Super
Sized
Kids

ALSO BY WALT LARIMORE:

10 Essentials of Highly Healthy People

The Highly Healthy Child

Why ADHD Doesn't Mean Disaster
(coauthored with Dennis Swanberg and Diane Passno)

Lintball Leo's Not-So-Stupid Questions About Your Body

God's Design for the Highly Healthy Child

God's Design for the Highly Healthy Teen

God's Design for the Highly Healthy Person

Alternative Medicine: The Christian Handbook
(coauthored with Dónal O'Mathúna)

*Bryson City Tales: Stories of a Doctor's First Year
of Practice in the Smoky Mountains*

*Bryson City Seasons: More Tales of a Doctor's Practice
in the Smoky Mountains*

Super Sized Kids

HOW TO RESCUE YOUR CHILD FROM THE OBESITY THREAT

WALT LARIMORE, MD
SHERRI FLYNT, MPH, RD, LD
with STEVE HALLIDAY

CENTER
STREET

NEW YORK BOSTON NASHVILLE

Center Street

Warner Books
Time Warner Book Group
1271 Avenue of the Americas, New York, NY 10020
Visit our Web site at www.twbookmark.com.

Center Street and the Center Street logo are trademarks of
Time Warner Book Group Inc.

Printed in the United States of America

First Edition: August 2005
10 9 8 7 6 5 4 3 2 1

Library of Congress Cataloging-in-Publication Data

Larimore, Walter L.
SuperSized kids : how to rescue your child from the obesity threat /
Walt Larimore, Sherri Flynt, and Steve Halliday.—1st ed.
p. cm.
Includes index.
ISBN 0-446-57760-X
1. Obesity in children—Popular works.   I. Flynt, Sherri.
II. Halliday, Steve, 1957–   III. Title.
RJ399.C6L27   2005
618.92'398—dc22   2005010518

To Barb and George: Your love, support, encouragement, and prayers carried us through this new adventure

ACKNOWLEDGMENTS

A book of this magnitude simply cannot be written without the support and labor of a large team of folks who believed in, encouraged, and enabled the massive effort required.

We feel grateful to the team at Florida Hospital for its assistance. The administrative support and encouragement of Don Jernigan, Des Cummings, Jr., Terry Newmyer, and Sy Saliba is gratefully acknowledged. We also benefited from the professionals who reviewed this book for accuracy. We made it our goal to create a book both trustworthy and evidence-based. To that end, the significant efforts of Dick Duerksen, Lenore Hodges, Ph.D., R.D., L.D., Paul Garrett, M.D., and Robert Quigley, M.D., are enthusiastically recognized; as is the valuable input of Dorlinda House, M.D., F.A.A.P., Naznin Dixit, M.D., D.M., Scott Brady, M.D., and the research team at the Florida Hospital Medical Library.

This book is the first in a series to be produced by Florida Hospital in Orlando. The series began in the imagination of a very creative, passionate, and energetic man. Without his and his assistant's endless encouragement and enthusiasm, this book would never have come to be. We extend our most special thanks to Todd Chobotar and Lillian Boyd. We are indebted to Lee Hough at Alive Communications, literary agent par excellence, who not only represents us professionally but has become a special friend. The efforts of these talented folks to put this resource into your hands cannot be overestimated. Thanks also to Rick Christian of Alive Communications for his wisdom and guidance. Thank you to Spencer Freeman for his wonderful photography work on the author photos and Paul Martin for his creative work on the graphics. We are grateful to Rolf Zettersten, Christina

Boys, and the entire team at Warner Faith and Center Street Publishers for their vision and labor in bringing this resource to you, our readers.

We also stand amazed at the incredible talent and gifts of Steve Halliday, our professional writing guide. He took our thoughts and vision, our research and practice experiences, our stories and passion, and combined a mountain of colors and hues into the final portrait you are about to enjoy. We hope you'll never forget the picture he helped us paint.

And now for a few very personal acknowledgments . . .

I am thankful for the opportunity to be involved in such an important project. Barb, you have my eternal thanks for your love, prayers, and support, as this book took me away from you more than either of us had planned. Thanks to Rolf, Todd, Lee, Christina, and Sherri for allowing me to work with you.

Walt Larimore, MD, DABFP
Monument, Colorado

I will never forget the experience of writing this book. I am grateful to the people who helped make it a reality. Shawn—for your support while I worked on this project. Lenore—for encouraging me to try something new. Ruth, Susan, and Meredith—thanks for lending your professional expertise. Dave—thanks for being such a trouper through all the long phone calls. Walt—it has been a pleasure. Max and Austin—for graciously allowing me to share part of your story. Mom, Dad, and Mike—your love and support have made me the person I am today. George—for enduring the long hours and our missed Sundays together without one complaint. I love you!

Sherri Flynt, MPH, RD, LD
Orlando, Florida

CONTENTS

INTRODUCTION

This book was written for moms and dads who want to raise their children to enjoy lives free from the ravages of obesity. To help you do this, we'll explore the latest research and share stories and experiences from patients and families who have struggled—and still struggle—with weight. Together, we will look at what it takes to save your children from the threat of obesity and offer you a series of simple, practical, and effective steps to get started.

There are five areas that we see as essential in raising children who have the knowledge and the power to avoid becoming or remaining SuperSized:

- Increased family involvement
- Adequate rest
- Reduced exposure to TV, computers, and video games
- Daily health-promoting activity
- Good nutrition

At first you might think that several of these factors have nothing to do with your children's weight. We want you to discover why they do.

We'll explore these areas in depth and even give you and your family a game plan for becoming a "healthy weight" family. But please remember that raising a healthy-weight child takes more than knowledge. It requires action—*your* action! Putting into practice the small steps we suggest in this book will get you on the road to saving your children from becoming (or remaining) SuperSized.

GETTING THE MOST OUT OF THIS BOOK

SuperSized Kids will assist you in one of the most important and difficult jobs you'll ever have—raising a healthy child. You can maximize the benefits of this book in at least three ways:

Option 1. Read through the book quickly to get an overview. Don't study; just skim through and learn. You might want to choose this option if you like to see the big picture, the overall view, before you decide where to begin. You can then read the book again more thoroughly or go straight to our eight-week plan in Appendix B and begin implementing some positive steps right away.

Option 2. Slowly read and study the book, doing the assessments and considering the "small step" suggestions as you go. This option will be most useful if you feel ready *today* to begin raising healthy-weight children. Be prepared to stop and incorporate each agreeable recommendation into your or your child's life. Or you can wait until you've finished the entire book and then use Appendix A or B to implement a plan for your family. Either way, be prepared to spend time meditating, studying, and learning. But give yourself time. When you're finished, the book should be dog-eared and worn—an effort well worth it!

Option 3. Before you read a word of the book, turn to Appendix A and assess your child's SuperSize status. This option is for those who want immediate help but don't have time to read the entire book. If you know of a problem in your home and you want quick relief, then this is the option for you. Once you identify particular problem areas, you will be directed to the part of the book most likely to help.

No matter which option you choose, you can use the eight-week action plan (Appendix B) to help you and your kids succeed in the battle ahead.

Getting involved as a family is crucial in the struggle against excess weight. So with any of these options, consider reviewing the information as a family. Maybe you could read a portion of a chapter every day with your kids and then as a family discuss what you've read.

USING A JOURNAL WHILE READING THIS BOOK

Purchase a new journal to use as you read this book. Journals with blank and lined pages are available at most bookstores. Write your name, your children's names, and the date you begin your journey on the first page. Keep your journal with this book and jot down your thoughts, feelings, and decisions as you read.

Why use a journal as you read this book? Because doing so can help motivate you and your family to make the changes you need to make to prevent or treat SuperSized Kids. By using a journal, you'll be able to decide not only what your family may want to do, but what you and your family can do. Try to make your observations and goals as specific as possible.

As you journal, you'll be able to review each principle and the action you're taking, as well as each goal you set. Be sure to choose a date by which you want to accomplish each goal. But remember, your family is a work in progress . . . so relax. Allow plenty of time to accomplish each goal. Remember, too, that making progress toward your goals—even if it feels slow—is much more important than setting goals you can't reach.

USING THE INTERNET

At times we recommend resources easily accessible via the Internet. We don't normally provide the Internet addresses for these sites, however, for two reasons: (1) Web addresses tend to change without notice, and (2) we might find better sites in the future. Therefore, Florida Hospital has assisted us in building an Internet site (www.SuperSizedKids.com) that you'll be able to visit at no cost. Here you'll find a list of the Internet sites we've recommended. By double-clicking on these listings, you'll be taken to the most up-to-date site for the information or health tool you need. We update this site as often as needed. In addition, blank food and activity pyramids, the eight-week plan (Appendix B), and the SuperSize assessment tool (Appendix A) are all available at www.SuperSizedKids.com for you to print and use.

So, if you're ready, let's get started. We'll begin by peering into the lives of some ordinary kids who struggle with today's SuperSizing.

PART ONE

The Coming Catastrophe

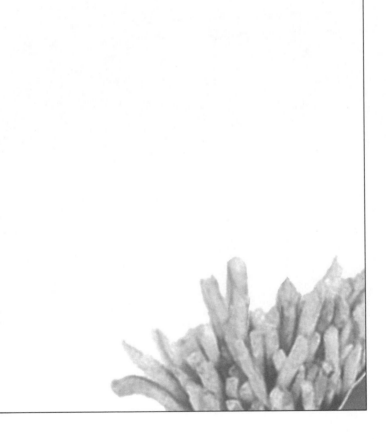

1

YOUNG FACES, ADULT PROBLEMS

He struggles to lift his foot, then his leg, over the frame of his bicycle. Sweat pours down his face as he accomplishes the task—easy for most people, daunting for Michael.[1] Out of breath, he sits for a moment to regain his strength. He may not like these short bike rides down the street and back, but he's heard countless times from his doctor that exercise is crucial to his losing weight and becoming healthier. And Michael needs to lose some pounds. A lot of pounds.

It's been two years since Michael was diagnosed with type 2 diabetes. A few months ago he landed in the hospital after his blood sugar levels rocketed out of control; there he learned that he suffered from a host of obesity-related health problems that threaten his life. To stay among the living, he needs to monitor his blood sugar four times a day, have blood tests frequently, remain under the care of several specialists, and receive regular insulin shots—all extremely expensive necessities.

Michael knows all about how obesity can ruin a person's life. It has ruined his.

Michael is seven years old.

"It's like a six-year-old going on sixty," says his doctor, a pediatric endocrinologist who, like all of us who care for children, increasingly treats young patients suffering from life-shortening ailments formerly seen only in men and women nearing retirement age. Today an exploding number of kids—many as young as six—suffer from an ugly range of deadly medical disorders, including diabetes, hypertension, kidney disease, and heart disease. According to the American Diabetes Association, the youngest documented victim of type 2 diabetes so far is a four-year-old Pima Indian.

"I'm afraid that if we don't do something now to prevent cases like these," says Michael's doctor, "this could be the generation with the shortest life span."

Unfortunately these cases aren't as rare as you might think. One of Walt Larimore's most memorable patients was three-year-old Sarah, whom he wrote about in *God's Design for a Highly Healthy Teen*. The first time Walt met Sarah she was sipping a baby bottle filled with Coke and was already obese, weighing forty-five pounds. Her mother tipped the scales at 250 pounds, and everyone in her family—father, siblings, aunts, and uncles—packed on at least one hundred pounds more than the recommended weight for his or her height. No one in the family exercised.

At age eight Sarah spent her first fear-filled nights in the hospital for diabetes; two years later she suffered from high blood pressure. Before long she had to deal with asthma, heart problems, and dozens of hospitalizations. When she was only fourteen years old, Sarah slipped into a diabetic coma and entered the hospital for the last time; there she died of a massive heart attack. Walt never felt lower in all his years of caring for adolescents.

PUTTING A FACE ON IT

The number of obese American children has skyrocketed in the last two decades, saddling these youngsters with an ugly host of disturbing and even lethal problems essentially unknown to their age group until the past few years. Without your care and caring as a parent, it's not only possible but likely that one or more of your children could slowly, almost imperceptibly at first, slide down this dangerous slope.

Food for Thought

In 2000, nearly twice as many kids were obese as compared to 1970.

Before we look at the statistics and facts of the obesity epidemic, let's look into the lives of real kids who are currently struggling with obesity. None of the three children you're about to meet have, as yet, plummeted to a physical condition anywhere near as alarming as that of Michael or Sarah. But they all face challenges with weight gain that are moving them in the same direction. Their stories also highlight many of the crucial issues that any successful approach to childhood obesity must first grasp, then tackle.

I'll Keep My Shirt On

Eleven-year-old Robert first started gaining an unhealthy amount of weight when he began taking oral steroids to help control his asthma. He was hospitalized for the first time at age seven and then again three years later.

Robert's mom grew very concerned when she found out that her son's blood sugar levels had risen to prediabetic stages. But rather than continue to just worry, she took immediate steps to deal with it. She realized that she needed to make changes in the way the entire family ate (see Chapter 5, "The Family Business"). "We all went on a diet," she declares. She eliminated all sugar and refined white flour from the household pantry. While Robert used to eat Frosted Flakes or a cinnamon-toast cereal for breakfast, now he gets a bran cereal that he loves and 2 percent milk. And how does he feel about that? Surprisingly he says, "I don't feel like having sugar that much any-more," though he admits it was hard to give up soft drinks and donuts.

Robert's eating challenges increase dramatically at school (see Chapter 11, "Be Part of the School Solution"). He usually eats at the school cafeteria, and for lunch often chooses pizza with a thick crust, hamburgers, hot dogs, or chicken nuggets—and, always, french fries. For a beverage he prefers milk or chocolate milk and sometimes orange juice. For dessert he likes various kinds of fruit (especially kiwifruit and strawberries), as well as brownies and cookies. He also admits to occasionally getting a candy bar from a vending cart.

Because of his asthma, Robert doesn't like to run a lot; his mom says running quickly makes him short of breath. During recess, he typically doesn't go out to play, but works on math problems instead. And when he gets home, everyone in his family goes for a walk, at least every other day.

Robert knows all of this is important to keep his weight down, and he also cooperates because of the way a slimmer physique makes him feel. He admits that his size made him feel "a little sad," and while few classmates called him fat or made fun of him because of his extra weight, at least one fourth grader did say nasty things about him and do insulting impressions of his appearance. "I don't want to be made fun of like that," Robert said, looking at the floor. Perhaps that's why Robert still doesn't like to take off his T-shirt when he goes swimming at the pool.

Food for Thought

"I don't want to be made fun of."

Robert

Robert, like most boys his age, likes video games. His parents allow him to play one "questionable" game, *Grand Theft Auto,* just once a week for an hour or so (see Chapter 7, "From Boob Tube to Mean Screen"). Sometimes Robert plays video games before breakfast. When he visits a friend's house after school or on the weekends, they often play basketball for a half hour and then go to the friend's room, where they look at game magazines and play Game Boy. Occasionally they might drink some water, but more often they down a few glasses of lemonade or slushies.

In our short interview Robert kept his head down and his lips pursed most of the time, but he's not afraid to look an adult in the eye and say what he thinks. And he also didn't shy away from telling us about a thirty-something friend of the family who suffers from diabetes—a friend who has only about three months to live.

"It's too late for him," Robert said softly.

"I Don't Know What Else to Do"

At birth Jimmy weighed a whopping twelve pounds. He tipped the scales at 150 pounds by age ten, and in the next couple of years he put on another twenty pounds. He's thirteen years old now, and within the last year a doctor told him that if he stayed on his current course, he'd be dead by age twenty-five.

So does Jimmy worry about his health? A little. His best friend's mom has diabetes and is "really big." And he also can't get out of his mind a recent scene. "I saw an old guy," he said, "four hundred pounds, who had to get an insulin shot. It's scary that my weight's going up again. I don't want to be like him."

But Jimmy's mom worries that he will be. "I think he will gain weight now," she said sadly. She can't help but think about a friend's granddaughter, a seventeen-year-old girl who weighs 350 pounds, wears size 42 pants, and at school has to use a handicapped desk. The girl rarely ventures outside of her house.

> *Food for Thought*
> "I have to do something, but I don't know what."
> Jimmy's mom

"We just don't know how to continue," she says. "I have to do something, but I don't know what. It feels like there are a thousand pieces out there, but I'm still looking for the pieces that match. I don't know what else to do." She feels deeply frustrated and isolated.

She feels especially alone since she and Jimmy's father got a divorce four years ago. Jimmy lives with his mom, but he's essentially a latchkey kid, because he stays at home alone much of the time due to her long work hours. She normally leaves home by 6:30 A.M. and often doesn't return until 9 P.M. When we met with her and Jimmy, she had just finished working a second job, from 4 P.M. the previous day until 8 A.M. the day of our interview.

Despite the long working hours, however, money remains very tight. Last year Jimmy had the funds to do some speed skating, which he loves (and which helps to keep his weight down), but this year that option has evaporated due to lack of money. So instead of switching to another form of exercise, he mostly stays home and watches TV (see Chapter 8, "Get Up, Get Out, Get Fun, Get Fit"). "It's easier to do things if you have money," he says with a glower toward his mom.

Jimmy doesn't get a lot of exercise, but he does look forward to gym class, he admits, because he loves to "sit and take roll." Once in a while he plays a little basketball and reports proudly that he can now run a lap around the school track within the set time limit; the first time he tried, it took him a quarter of an hour.

Eating the right things is a challenge for both Jimmy and his mom (see Chapter 9, "Overfed and Undernourished"). For breakfast that morning she said she had a bowl of spaghetti. And she figures that Jimmy goes through about ten two-liter bottles of soda pop a week (and not the diet stuff). She also admits that at work the night before, she herself drank three bottles of soda. Jimmy says that he might drink more water if he didn't have to boil the apartment tap water to make it safe. "To buy water takes money," he says.

Jimmy doesn't have a regular doctor or medical insurance and hasn't had an appointment with a physician since he got the ominous warning about his weight. "Can I afford a doctor's visit for fifteen minutes?" his mom asks, then answers her own question: "No, I cannot!" Still, she says she hopes to take Jimmy back to the doctor before school starts in the fall.

Jimmy may not have a regular doctor, but a friend of his recently introduced him to the Great Physician. "My friend invited me to go to church with him," Jimmy reported with a smile. "I wrote down two numbers from the Bible on my shoe."

On the tongue of his left sneaker he shows us the words from Psalm 27:1, scrawled in ballpoint pen: "The Lord is my light and salvation—whom shall I fear?" But Jimmy's mom shakes her head disapprovingly and makes it clear she wants nothing to do with "religion." So Jimmy quickly drops his head and the subject.

Last year Jimmy's grandmother grew concerned over his weight gain and forced her grandson to walk five miles a day. He soon lost twenty-five pounds, but since then has put most of it back on. "I have to apply myself" to reach a healthier weight, Jimmy says, but he has no real plan to do so. Still, he has hope.

"Rocky came out victorious," he said, recalling the fictional Hollywood boxer. "Hopefully I can end up on top."

Food for Thought

"Hopefully I can end up on top."

Jimmy

Like Parents, Like Daughter?

Fourteen-year-old Angel arrived for her interview accompanied by her father, a man weighing in excess of four hundred pounds, who says simply, "I've always been big." Angel's mom, recently diagnosed with diabetes, is also very large and has been in and out of the hospital for weight-related maladies more than twenty times. Angel's own excess weight bothers her—"No one really understands," she says—but so far, she's had limited success in keeping off the extra pounds.

Recently Angel did join a gym at Florida Hospital's diabetes center, along with her mom (her dad is awaiting a medical clearance to join). A few times a week she does sit-ups there and uses the stationary bike and treadmill, usually for about fifteen minutes, but hardly breaks a sweat. Angel hates running and describes her school's "three-lap Thursdays" as "horrible." She has tried to get moving to an old exercise video, but she found it boring and says that "it felt like a time warp back to the eighties."

These days Angel gets most of her exercise in band class (it counts at her school as physical education). In middle school she tried out for the volleyball team but didn't make it, and since then she's stuck almost exclusively with band. During the last marching season she dropped a couple of dress sizes, but in the off-season she gained back most of the pounds she had lost. Other than marching band and the very light workouts at the gym, she doesn't get a lot of exercise. She admits to watching a lot of TV and often sits in front of the computer.

Angel doesn't eat breakfast and only rarely eats lunch. She says she tried to eat breakfast when she started riding the bus to school, but since she gets carsick easily, she doesn't bother with breakfast anymore. And because there's "lots of competition at lunchtime" at her school (students are allowed about half an hour to eat), she usually doesn't eat then, either. Occasionally she'll eat in the band room: a candy bar, some chips, a few cheesy crackers, a piece of pizza, and a soda or two.

Normally Angel gets home from school about 3:15. By then she's very hungry, so she picks up something quick to eat—what she calls a grab-and-run snack—usually at Wendy's: maybe a burger and fries, or two chicken sandwiches and fries.

For dinner Angel often fixes her own meal: fries, a whole chicken slathered with ranch dressing and ketchup, frozen corn. She likes fried chicken better than baked chicken, and she also loves steak. Her dad says her favorite restaurant features what he calls huge portions.

Angel doesn't like fruit or vegetables; she hasn't eaten an apple since elementary school. Why not? "I had allergies to fruit juices when I was a baby," she explains.

Still, she says she's willing to do "whatever it takes" to make some changes in her diet. She used to drink four or five bottles a day of regular soda pop; now she's down to about two a day. (When her mom and dad first met, her mother drank the equivalent of a six-pack of soda every day. Now Mom is down to one or two diet soft drinks a day.)

And what has Angel learned so far? In sixth and seventh grades she gained a lot of weight, "but I got so that I didn't care," she said. In eighth grade she decided to do something about her weight and enjoyed some success—but staying with it is hard.

ON TO THE NUMBERS

Too many of our kids are fat and getting fatter. In some areas of the country up to 40 percent of the children are obese or extremely overweight. We personally know one obese toddler who got stuck in his high chair. We know a fourteen-year-old who collapsed a chair at a restaurant just by sitting down; the child weighs almost three hundred pounds. Doctors across the nation continue to report dangerously high blood pressure and severe vascular changes in boys and girls as young as six years old.

Think about that for a moment. If we're pushing the onset of diabetes and heart disease to age five or six—remember Michael?—the affected child's parents may see terrible health complications striking that child *within their own lifetimes.*

We simply have to face the truth: SuperSized Kids are *not* normal—their overweight status is a potential killer. Obese kids aren't merely chubby; they're facing a real and brutal health crisis. And if we don't do something *now* to help them get back on the right track, the story may end on a grim note.

Sorry to say, the numbers don't lie. You may find the next chapter hard to read—it's packed with cold, hard statistics and study findings that could make you wince—but please stick with it. Take a deep breath, prepare yourself for a short but bumpy ride, and plunge in. When we say obesity *crisis* we really mean it. And we're not alone.

2

THE PERFECT STORM

More and more of America's kids are overweight. And unless we do something now, America itself may not have much of a future.

Shocked researchers have found, for example, that more than 40 percent of New York City public school students are overweight, and nearly one-quarter are obese, meaning their health is significantly threatened. Even our youngest children are in trouble. New research shows that 22 percent of two- to four-year-olds participating in a New York City nutrition program are overweight, and another 18 percent are dangerously close to becoming so.[1]

These worrisome findings echo those of a highly publicized study released in June 2004 demonstrating that 40 percent of children in rural Arkansas are also overweight or obese. "We need to sound an alarm, not only for Arkansas but for the entire country," said Dr. Joe Thompson, director of the Arkansas Center for Health Improvement.[2]

Food for Thought

"We need to sound an alarm . . . for the entire country!"

Dr. Joe Thompson
Director, Arkansas Center
for Health Improvement

Think that sounds overblown? It's really not. A growing number of health care experts have called the childhood obesity epidemic a disaster in the making for the nation's economy and health care system. But when that looming crisis combines with two other major developments—the retirement of the baby boom generation and the serious fiscal woes of both Medicare and the Social Security system— it has all the makings of a perfect storm: a massive collision of rampaging fronts with the power to cause staggering damage.

A KILLER EPIDEMIC

We really ought to listen when leading health care authorities from all over the nation issue urgent warnings that sound frighteningly similar.

- "We have an epidemic of obesity in the United States and it's only getting worse," said U.S. Surgeon General Richard Carmona. "We are seeing Generation Y grow into Generation XL, and this weight gain has long-term health consequences."[3]
- "We've never had a population like this before," said Naomi Neufeld, a pediatric endocrinologist and director of KidShape, a nonprofit weight-loss program. "Children who are overweight are 20 percent to 30 percent heavier now than they were even ten years ago. We can't even imagine the medical costs we will be seeing in the future. It feels like Armageddon."[4]
- "This is tragic," said Dr. Julie Gerberding, director of the federal Centers for Disease Control and Prevention (CDC). "Obesity has got to be job No. 1 for us in terms of chronic diseases."[5]
- According to the National Academy of Sciences, obesity health care costs for children more than tripled in twenty years: from $35 million a year in 1979 to $127 million a year in 1999.[6]

Food for Thought

According to Emory University researchers, more than a quarter of the phenomenal growth in health care spending over the past fifteen years is attributable to obesity.[7]

Failure to stem the obesity epidemic in our kids will cost each of us, our children, and our children's children in ways we can't even begin to imagine. In 2000, for example, U.S. airlines had to spend $275 million to burn 350 million more gallons of fuel than expected, just to carry the additional weight of fat Americans![8] Southwest Airlines recently responded to the extra costs by charging obese passengers for two tickets; other airlines were expected to follow suit.

One major consequence of the scourge of childhood obesity has already become abundantly clear. In 2000 the nation suffered more than 300,000 obesity-related fatalities, making obesity one of the leading causes of preventable deaths. In fact, according to the CDC, if the current trend is not reversed (and we have no indication that it is losing steam), obesity will soon become the nation's number one cause of preventable death.

"Obesity is not a superficial question of appearance," warned Dr. Gerald Hass, physician in chief at the South End Community Health Center in Boston. "It is the number one health crisis facing inner-city children—one that will shorten their lives and cost society billions of dollars if we don't start working seriously toward solutions."[9]

Food for Thought

"It's dead wrong to write off weight problems as somebody else's personal problem. We are all paying the epidemic's costs. More than 100,000 stomach-reduction operations take place annually, with insurance companies—meaning all policyholders—under intense pressure to pick up the tab."

New York Daily News
November 30, 2004

Hass, a dedicated pediatrician who has worked closely with children for more than three decades, declared:

Obesity leads these children to heart disease, hypertension, respiratory ailments, orthopedic problems, and diabetes. The skyrocketing rate of obesity among lower income children is also dramatically reducing the quality of these young lives. I see obese children and teens every day. As their pediatrician, I see the depression and hopelessness that go hand-in-hand with the physical problems.

The problem is relatively new and rapidly worsening. Thirty-three years ago, when I began treating the children of the South End and Lower Roxbury, I was not confronted with 300-pound fourteen-year-olds. We worried about chicken pox and measles in children, but not Type II diabetes in teens.

Now, a shocking 40 percent of our 8,000 pediatric patients at the South End Community Health Center are clinically obese. On a recent Friday, 75 percent of the children I saw were obese.[10]

Hass reacts to this gathering storm by urging immediate action on a number of fronts. He also sharply challenges those who "say that 'personal responsibility' should drive better health behavior . . . That is a hard argument to make in the face of a depressed, obese child whose health is failing, who has no safe place to exercise, and is under siege by adults selling him salt, fat, sugar, and a shorter, sadder life. As adults, we have an obligation to do better."[11]

Before we can do better, however, we have to understand what all these experts are talking about. This crisis they're practically shouting themselves hoarse over—what is it? What does it look like? How close is it?

THE SCOPE OF THE EPIDEMIC

A report issued in October 2002 by the CDC declared that more than 15 percent of American children aged six to nineteen were overweight—a whopping *200 percent* increase over the previous three decades. And the news is considerably worse for Mexican

Americans and non-Hispanic blacks: More than 23 percent of children aged twelve to nineteen in both groups were considered clinically overweight[12]—a startling 120 percent increase just from 1986 to 1998.[13]

And still, our children get bigger. One report found that more than 10 percent of U.S. children two through five years old are *already* overweight. By age ten many of these children will have become obese, with early symptoms of diabetes. In one study almost 40 percent of children were considered obese before the age of six; children as young as four had abnormally high insulin levels (a risk factor for diabetes); and 13 percent of children showed high cholesterol levels.[14]

Even in sunny, supposedly health-conscious California nearly 40 percent of children are considered physically unfit, while more than 25 percent are overweight, according to a report by the California Center for Public Health Advocacy.

"Forget the image of granola-loving Californians who love to surf, bike, or play beach volleyball," said Joanne Ikeda, codirector of the Center for Weight and Health and cooperative extension specialist at the University of California at Berkeley's College of Natural Resources. "When it comes to the prevalence of child obesity, California outpaces the national average."[15]

Unfortunately this epidemic is not just an issue in the United States. Researchers found that while two-thirds of Great Britain's schoolchildren were overweight or obese, their parents did not believe it. A third of obese girls and half of the obese boys were rated by their parents as weighing "about right." Moreover, one-third of mothers and half the fathers who were either overweight or obese rated themselves "about right." Researcher Alison Jeffery said, "When the weight that physicians know to be hazardously overweight is considered normal weight by the general public, major health problems are on the horizon." She added, "When parents do not recognize overweight and obesity in their children—as up to three-quarters of the parents in our survey did not—we are missing critical partners in our effort to halt a developing epidemic."[16]

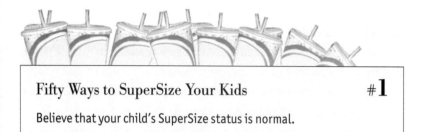

Fifty Ways to SuperSize Your Kids   #1

Believe that your child's SuperSize status is normal.

FROM OBESE CHILDREN TO OBESE ADULTS

An obese child tends to become an obese adult—and that makes for significant trouble.

Recent research suggests that obese teenagers have a dramatically increased risk of dying by the time they reach middle age. One study found that overweight teenagers had a mortality rate thirty to forty times higher than teens of normal weight. And can you guess the average age of death for adults who were obese as adolescents? Not sixty. Not fifty-five. Not even fifty. Children in the study who were obese as teens died as adults at the average age of forty-six.[17]

Dead by age forty-six! How's that for a frightening consequence of childhood obesity?

Food for Thought

Obesity is clearly associated with large decreases in life expectancy. That means it's a killer lying in wait for our kids.

Another report, titled "Years of Life Lost Due to Obesity," found that, depending upon the sex and race of the individual, obesity lowers life expectancy *from eight to twenty years*! Even more significant, perhaps, the report pointed out that "obesity significantly impairs quality of life, arguably a more potent marker of the effect of obesity because quality-of-life deficits are experienced in the moment rather than anticipated sometime in the future."[18] In other words, while you can tell yourself that everyone has to die someday, it's not so easy to convince yourself that your many extra pounds are worth the intense misery and pain they cause you every waking moment of every day.

And just in case you missed the point, hear the conclusion of one more study: "Severely obese children and adolescents have lower health-related quality of life than children and adolescents who are healthy, and *similar quality of life as those diagnosed as having cancer*" (italics added).[19]

Food for Thought

Severely obese kids have a quality of life similar to that of children who have cancer.

Obesity in childhood has a strong tendency to persist into adulthood, a tendency that rises dramatically in homes with at least one obese parent.[20] Why is this important? There are at least two reasons.

First, in times past, many physicians tended to look at childhood obesity as little more than a glitch in appearance—the poor kid might look fat and have to take a little ribbing, but he or she would soon grow out of it. The problem with this idea? It simply isn't true. Overweight and obese children tend to become overweight and obese adults, with all the health problems associated with packing on far too many pounds.

Food for Thought

Obesity has become one of the leading causes of preventable death in the United States.

Once and for all, let's get this straight: Childhood obesity is not primarily an issue of *appearance*. That's why the authors of one medical review urged their colleagues to see the SuperSized Kids problem as a major cause of ill health in *both* children and adults.[21]

And that leads us to the second reason why we must attack childhood obesity *now*. While obese children tend to become obese adults who suffer all the related health problems, the fact is, we are beginning to see children who, *as children*, are suffering from the same terrible maladies that have long afflicted their portly elders.

Their terrible plight calls to mind a prophetic warning sounded to an adult audience more than two decades ago by cultural observer Ralph Winter:

> The underdeveloped societies suffer from one set of diseases: tuberculosis, malnutrition, pneumonia, parasites, typhoid, cholera, typhus, etc. Affluent America has virtually invented a whole new set of diseases: obesity, arteriosclerosis, heart disease, stroke, lung cancer, venereal disease, cirrhosis of the liver, drug addiction, alcoholism, divorce, battered children, suicide, murder. Take your choice. Laborsaving machines have turned out to be body-killing devices. Our affluence has allowed both mobility and isolation of the nuclear family, and as a result our divorce courts, our prisons and our mental institutions are flooded.[22]

THE PRESENT-DAY CONSEQUENCES OF CHILDHOOD OBESITY

If you don't think it hurts our kids to pack on those extra pounds, you had better think again. All kinds of rigorous scientific studies have confirmed the appalling current-day results of childhood obesity on our kids. Consider just a few of them:

Psychological consequences. Obese children are more likely to suffer psychological or psychiatric problems than nonobese children, and obesity is often associated with low self-esteem and behavioral problems.[23] In addition, obese children are more likely to bully other children or to be bullied.[24]

Social and economic consequences. Obese children moving into their late teens and early twenties tend to be financially poorer and socially less well connected than their normal-weight peers.

Cardiovascular consequences. Obese children tend to have high blood pressure, higher "bad" cholesterol, excessive blood sugar, and other related problems "similar to those well known in adults."[25] They are more prone to a cluster of symptoms known as metabolic syndrome, which often precedes cardiovascular disease and type 2 diabetes.[26] Some obese children as young as seven years old already have the beginnings of artery disease.[27] In addition, extremely obese youngsters may be at serious risk for heart attacks. And the heavier the child, the higher the risk.[28]

Respiratory consequences. Obese children tend to develop asthma at a higher rate than other children, and those who already suffer from asthma tend to develop more serious cases.[29] One study found that asthma cases complicated by obesity rose 40 percent.[30] Researchers in Hong Kong found that obese children are 20 percent more likely to have signs of sleep apnea than normal-weight children—important because sleep apnea has been linked to poor concentration and attention problems[31] (and has increased fivefold since 1979 in obese children).

Surgery. Bariatric surgery—formerly a rare procedure to reduce the size of the stomach—is performed with increasing frequency each year in the United States and is becoming more popular among teens. More than 45,000 patients had some type of surgery for obesity in 2001, 65,000 in 2002, and more than 100,000 in 2003. Exponential increase is expected over the next ten years, along with a growing number of facilities offering these services.[32]

Cancer consequences. One British study claims that overweight children are at increased risk of cancer later in life. The risk of adulthood cancer increased by 9 percent for every standard increment in childhood body mass index (BMI). No other factors—such as socioeconomic status, body composition, energy intake during childhood, or birth order—seemed to have this effect.[33]

Liver damage. A serious condition known as nonalcoholic fatty liver now afflicts up to 52 percent of obese children.[34] This condition resembles alcoholic liver disease but occurs with little or no alcohol intake. Fat accumulates in the liver, inflammation occurs, and the liver becomes damaged. If not detected and treated, nonalcoholic fatty liver can lead to permanent liver damage.

Orthopedic consequences. People who suffer from obesity often have problems with their feet, caused by carrying around too much weight.

Food for Thought

Doctors now believe that 10 percent to 20 percent of all cancers are related to obesity; by preventing obesity early in life, it appears that many of these cancers can be avoided.

Arguably the most chilling consequence of childhood obesity is the renaming of an old disease. In the past, type 1 diabetes was known as juvenile diabetes, and it's bad enough that obese children have more than a twofold risk of developing it as compared to normal children. But what used to be called adult-onset diabetes is now commonly referred to as type 2 (or non-insulin-dependent) diabetes. Why the name change? Because so many kids have it. During the past eight years the number of children diagnosed with type 2 diabetes has risen tenfold.[35]

Walt didn't see his first case of type 2 diabetes in a child until the late eighties, after he had been a physician for more than ten years. Apparently other physicians have had a similar experience. "Until recently, type 2 diabetes was rare in kids," said Dr. Christopher Still, a weight-control specialist. "Now it accounts for 40 percent to 50 percent of the diabetes among children."[36]

Type 2 diabetes puts children at risk for a smorgasbord of adult ailments, including kidney failure, cardiovascular disease, nerve damage, and blindness. If current estimates prove to be accurate, by the year 2050, 45 million to 50 million U.S. residents could have type 2 diabetes. And we're already well on our way: In the past ten years the number of diagnosed cases of diabetes has risen by nearly half, reaching 11 million in 2000.[37]

It's hard to imagine more severe consequences.

Or is it?

THE BABY BOOM RETIRES

The post–World War II generation known as the baby boom (those born from 1946 to 1964) expanded the U.S. population by about 77 million. As of 2003, boomers represented about 27.5 percent of the total U.S. population.

The oldest members of this group—the largest such group in American history—will start reaching normal retirement age in the next few years. As they do, they will begin calling on the health care system (including the already financially troubled Medicare) with greater frequency, to address the physical problems that accompany aging.

But what happens if, at the same time the baby boomers start drawing more heavily on the resources of the nation's health care system, tens of millions of obese-children-turned-obese-young-people also start drawing heavily on the health care system? What happens when these ailing twenty-somethings flood the country's clinics and hospitals with a range of serious diseases, from kidney failure to coronary collapse? How does the national health care system cope with the largest group of retirees in history at the same time that it must treat the largest group of ailing young people in history? It's a frightening thought.

But it gets worse.

COULD SUPERSIZED KIDS WRECK SOCIAL SECURITY AND MEDICARE?

For the past thirty years the sheer size of the baby boom generation has largely determined the size and age composition of the nation's labor force. In 1978 baby boomers (then aged fifteen to thirty-two) made up about 45 percent of the labor force. By 2008, workers aged forty-five and older will make up 40 percent of the labor force (as opposed to 33 percent in 1998). And when they begin to retire en masse, they'll leave a big hole in the worker pool. In fact, after 2008, "as more and more baby-boomers reach retirement age, the impact of their retirements will continue to grow."[38]

The need for more workers will be especially felt in educational services (teachers, administrators, counselors, etc.), the transportation industry (rail, bus, air, etc.), the health services industry (registered nurses, licensed practical nurses, registered dietitians, medical doctors, etc.), and the construction industry.

In the decade following 2008, however, the effects will grow even more dramatically. "By 2018, all but the youngest baby-boomers will be of retirement age. Aggravating the situation is a much smaller pool of workers immediately following the baby-boomers."[39]

So will this cause a labor force collapse in twenty years? Experts hope not, pointing to several "encouraging signs" that may help the nation to avoid such a catastrophic worker shortage, including large numbers of baby boomers delaying their retirement and an increasing number of immigrants.[40]

But what happens to America's future labor force if millions of obese young people are too sick to hold down steady jobs? What happens if a significant portion of an entire generation gets so fat that instead of reporting to work every morning, these obese men and women lie in oversized, structurally reinforced beds, hooked up to oxygen tanks, where they struggle to breathe from dawn to dusk? What happens then?

The Social Security system already includes the following lines in its mailed statements to program participants: "Without changes, by 2042 the Social Security Trust Fund will be exhausted. By then, the number of Americans 65 or older is expected to have doubled. There won't be enough younger people working to pay all of the benefits owed to those who are retiring."[41]

Is "collapse" too strong a word?

Food for Thought

"Every month the Social Security Administration pays $77 million to citizens whose disability is obesity-related."

New York Daily News
November 30, 2004

Federal Reserve Chairman Alan Greenspan has warned that the United States "will eventually have no choice but to make significant structural adjustments in the major retirement programs," a clear nod to future cuts in Social Security benefits.[42] Why? As Tim Penny, chairman of the national advisory board of For Our Grandchildren (a Social Security education program), says:

> The baby-boom generation is twice as large as the current crop of retirees—and soon there will not be enough paying workers to finance the program. The numbers are relentless. The most recent Social Security trustees' report calculates that by 2018, payroll taxes will be insufficient to cover annual Social Security benefits. At present, there are approximately 3½ workers for every retiree. But by 2030, when baby boomers are fully retired, there will be only two workers per retiree. Clearly, something has to give.[43]

If we don't avert this epidemic, not only will we see fewer workers and reduced tax income, but dramatically increased medical costs could threaten the health of the Medicare system. In late 2004 a chilling report in the prestigious *Journal of the American Medical Associa-*

tion declared that the more men and women weighed in middle age, the more Medicare charges they racked up—nearly double, in fact.[44] Is it possible that the obesity tsunami could end up sinking Social Security *and* Medicare and flood our health care industry in a sea of flab-related costs that could bankrupt us all? Again, to quote Mr. Penny, something has to give.

Something has to give, all right. But what's "giving out" at this very moment is the health of America's children. Keep this in mind: As gloomy as these predictions by Greenspan and Penny sound, they do not even acknowledge the very real possibility that *millions* of the young workers they're counting on for the future may not be able to work at all! Far from contributing financially to a teetering federal retirement program, these desperately ill young people will instead be trying to draw upon disability benefits to help cover the stratospheric cost of their many obesity-caused diseases.

What would happen then? It looks to us like nothing short of a perfect storm.

DO STATISTICS LIE?

"Now, hold on!" you may say. "Things can't possibly be as dark as all that. You can get statistics to say anything you want. You're just trying to scare me."

You know what? You're half right.

Oh, you're wrong about the statistics we've cited; we haven't manipulated them, nor have we reached conclusions at odds with the vast majority of other experts who see the very crisis we've just described.

But you're right about the "scare" part. We really do want to scare you—if that's what it takes to get you to come to grips with the crisis barreling down on our heads. Fear is a good thing if it causes us to sit up and take action against a very real evil that, left unopposed, would destroy us.

We've already spent enough time ignoring the childhood obesity epidemic. It's time we did something about it.

3

HOW DID WE GET INTO THIS MESS?

Don't look now, but someone has been busy SuperSizing your world.

At Disney's theme parks, engineers have enlarged ride turnstiles.

In emergency rooms and operating rooms across the country, patient gurneys and operating tables have grown bigger and been reinforced to handle wider and heavier bodies.

Ambulances now carry SuperSized stretchers.

Mattress companies have begun advertising beds that can bear up under thousand-pound loads.

Doctors at Massachusetts General Hospital in Boston have complained that obese patients are overwhelming their imaging machines and making it increasingly harder to peer inside. One researcher, Raul Uppot, suggested that equipment makers "need to think about design changes and technological advancements to obtain quality imaging in larger patients."[1]

The 2003 Oscar-nominated animated feature *The Triplets of Belleville* portrayed Americans as virtual land whales—swaying, sweating mountains of lard.

How did this happen? How did we get so heavy and so obsessed with such terrible nutrition choices? And how did our kids follow suit so quickly?

While we could cite dozens of factors to help explain the obesity epidemic now threatening the country, our unprecedented national weight gain essentially comes down to three things:

1. We're eating too many calories and too much of the wrong kinds of food.
2. We're moving less.
3. We're getting less sleep than we need.

And so are our kids.

On average we eat almost three hundred calories more per day and burn about three hundred calories less a day than we did twenty years ago. And where do those six hundred extra calories go? Our bodies store them as fat. When you consider that an additional one hundred calories a day can mean an extra ten pounds a year, it's not hard to see how our kids can so easily gain an unhealthful thirty pounds or more!

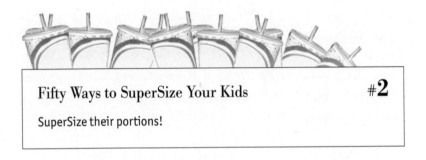

Fifty Ways to SuperSize Your Kids   #2

SuperSize their portions!

WE'RE EATING MORE . . . AND WORSE

Just as dozens of reasons can help to explain our ballooning waist-lines, so several factors help to make clear why we're eating more. Let's consider a few of the most prominent reasons.

SuperSized Portions

You probably haven't noticed it, but portion sizes have grown tremen-dously over the years, especially since the 1970s. A 2003 report in the *Journal of the American Medical Association* showed how the obesity epidemic has coincided with a marked increase in food portion sizes, particularly in fast-food restaurants. Consider these examples:

- The serving size of an average soft drink increased from 13 ounces (144 calories) in 1977 to almost 20 ounces (with fifteen teaspoons of sugar and 250 calories) in 1998.
- Cheeseburgers grew from 5.8 ounces (397 calories) in 1977 to 7.3 ounces (533 calories) in 1998.
- Salty snacks grew from 1 ounce (132 calories) in 1977 to 1.6 ounces (225 calories) in 1998.[2]

Go back a little further in time, and you'll see an even greater size disparity. In 1900, the average Hershey bar came in a 2-ounce package (297 calories); by 2004 it had grown to 7 ounces (1,000 calories). In 1916 the only Coke you could buy came in a 6.5-fluid-ounce bottle (79 calories); by 2004 the average serving size had risen to 16 fluid ounces (194 calories). In the 1950s moviegoers could buy about a 3-cup serving of popcorn (174 calories); by 2004 they were gobbling a 21-cup heavily buttered serving (1,700 calories). In 1954 an average Burger King hamburger weighed in at 2.8 ounces (202 calories); by 2004 it had jumped to 4.3 ounces (310 calories). In 1955 patrons got a 2.4-ounce serving of McDonald's fries (210 calories); in 2004 this had jumped to 7 ounces (610 calories).[3]

One-fourth of the U.S. population—that's 70 million of us—step inside the doors of a fast-food restaurant *every day*. So why should it surprise anyone that probably half of our children are chowing down on fast food every day?

These days a single fast-food meal can amount to an entire day's caloric intake for an adult—and for children that same meal could

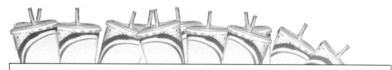

Fifty Ways to SuperSize Your Kids   #3

Let your kids eat frequently at fast-food restaurants.

SuperSized Portions
Then and Now

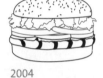

1954
2.8 oz
202 calories

2004
4.3 oz
310 calories

Hamburger

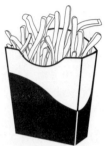

1955
2.4 oz
210 calories

2004
7 oz
610 calories

Fries

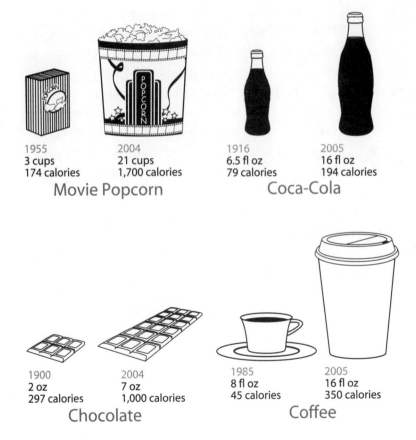

1955
3 cups
174 calories

2004
21 cups
1,700 calories

Movie Popcorn

1916
6.5 fl oz
79 calories

2005
16 fl oz
194 calories

Coca-Cola

1900
2 oz
297 calories

2004
7 oz
1,000 calories

Chocolate

1985
8 fl oz
45 calories

2005
16 fl oz
350 calories

Coffee

translate to *two* days' worth of calories. Even three pieces of pizza can exceed 1,600 calories and 80 grams of fat. That's an amazing amount of calories for one meal, and it doesn't even include dessert or the soda that most kids drink with it.

It ought to shock us to see just how big portion sizes have grown. Is it any wonder our kids are getting huge?

Increased Fast-Food and Soda Consumption

Almost one-third of American kids aged four to nineteen will eat today at a fast-food place, a fivefold increase since 1970. On average they will eat 187 more calories per day than those who refrain from fast food, and they will ingest more fats, sugars, and carbohydrates. As a result, they will pack on about an extra six pounds per year, according to one study.[4] That's appalling, of course, but the alarming news doesn't stop there. Some researchers contend that eating fast foods can become addictive. "New and potentially explosive findings on the biological effects of fast food suggest that eating yourself into obesity isn't simply down to a lack of self-control," said one scientist. As body fat increases, people appear to become increasingly insensitive to hormones that help to control their eating.[5] The more fast food you eat, the less you may feel like you're eating.

Most of us who frequent fast-food places also buy soft drinks there—and researchers at the University of North Carolina School of Public Health say that, more than anything else, it's these sugar-laden drinks that make us fat. "If we are going to consume more beverages, we are going to gain weight," said lead author Dr. Barry Popkin.

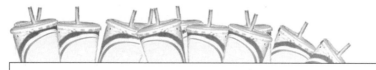

Fifty Ways to SuperSize Your Kids   #4

Give your kids lots of soft drinks!

And who gulps down the most soft drinks? Consumers between the ages of ten and thirty. "That's the time when it's even scarier, when we get our bone density, when we need milk and need many of the foods that have nutrients, not just nothing—which is what sugar has," Popkin declared. "Sugar has calories to make us fat with no other benefit."

Most soft drinks contain something called high-fructose corn syrup, a cheap sweetener discovered in the early 1970s. Over the past fifteen years the nation's consumption of this substance has grown by 250 percent; some experts estimate that we get as much as 9 percent of our daily calories from fructose. But researchers at the University of Michigan have concluded that fructose in high levels elevates dangerous triglycerides by as much as 32 percent and slows down the body's fat burning and storage system. Result? Weight gain.

Reduction of Family Meals

In many homes the family meal has gone the way of the dinosaur. Most families simply don't eat together as they used to. And that tends to pack on the pounds.

Think of it like this. A lot of restaurants, in an effort to lure you back or to keep you happy while waiting for your entrée, offer free chips or bread before the meal. You come in hungry, consume lots of free food, and then before your stomach has the time to tell your brain it's full, your oversized meal arrives and you eat the whole thing. We tend to eat the food in front of us, and many studies have shown that this holds true for children as well. If it's sitting there, we eat it.

In addition, when we eat out, we tend to eat faster. At home we eat more slowly and talk about the events of the day—and when we eat more slowly, we almost always eat less. Why? For one thing, a delay occurs between the time we ingest something and the time we start to feel satisfied. It takes about twenty-five to thirty minutes before we start to feel full. So when we eat more quickly, we are likely to eat more before this feeling of fullness hits.

Last, food prepared at home tends to be more healthful than food prepared in a restaurant. Eating out not only increases the portion size of our food but also reduces, for example, the number of fruits and vegetables we eat.

Reduction of Breakfast

Children don't eat breakfast like they once did, and children who don't eat breakfast have a strong tendency to enter a spiral of weight gain that ends in obesity. We'll say more about this later (Chapter 10, "Gearing Up for Healthful Family Meals"), but for now it's enough to say that a reduction in breakfast has been associated with an increase in childhood obesity.

Hectic Schedules

Hectic schedules—on the part of both parents and kids—have a nasty way of leading to excess pounds. They produce a double whammy: fewer healthful meals and less time for exercise. Sherri Flynt, who has been a registered dietitian for twenty years and currently works as the manager for the Center of Nutritional Excellence at Florida Hospital in Orlando, says that many parents tell her their kids get home early from school, while they themselves get home late from work. They don't want their children running around outside without them home, and children left home alone will gobble up snacks, healthful or unhealthful. So how do they occupy themselves while locked up inside, unable to go out and play? What takes their time? Video games, TV, the computer, and, yes, snacks.

Increasingly we hear child health experts say that wise parents must limit the number of their children's organized extracurricular group activities, choosing only the most beneficial for each child. Therefore, they should choose one sport that the child likes (instead of two), along with a more intellectual activity, such as violin or piano, and a spiritual activity, such as attending a church youth group. They should *not* opt for violin *and* cello *and* piano *and* soccer *and* track *and* the youth group *and* scouting. Such a hectic schedule runs both the child and the parent ragged and fills their days with far too many activities—as well as increasing the number of opportunities for unwanted weight gain.

Unhealthy Food at School

We'll talk more about this later (Chapter 11, "Be Part of the School Solution"), but many kids today put on weight, in part, because of what they eat in school. In the cafeteria they feast largely on a diet of burgers, hot dogs, pizza, fries, chips, and soda, and wrinkle their noses at more healthful options (so before long the school doesn't offer them). And maybe they carry around some extra change for a couple of candy bars or sodas or other snacks from school vending machines or carts. Pretty soon the pounds start adding up.

Fewer Healthy Food Choices in the Inner City

Kids in some inner cities have a tough time even getting their hands on healthful foods because over the years many large grocery stores have abandoned their neighborhoods. Fast-food outlets or convenience stores have moved in, offering tasty but highly processed fatty and sugary foods. To combat this problem, cities like Philadelphia have begun programs to try to entice grocery stores back to the inner city. (We'll talk more about what communities can do in Chapter 12, "Bring Unity to the Community.")

WE'RE EXERCISING LESS

The only part of our bodies that moves more than it used to is our mouths. We just don't get the exercise that we once did. And neither do our kids. Why? Let's look at some major changes in our society and our culture that have taken place over the past few decades.

Suburbanization of America

As large numbers of families started migrating to the suburbs after World War II, communities became more sprawling. As a result, people had to travel farther to shop, including for their groceries. So suburbanites learned to hop into their cars to get food. Many of us therefore get very little exercise, compared to food shoppers of even a few decades ago. Suburbanization has led to less walking and more car driving.

And what's so bad with that? Nothing, if you want to get fat.

A study published in 2004 in the *American Journal of Preventive Medicine* surveyed 10,500 metro Atlanta residents, tracking their travel behavior and measuring each participant's height and weight. It turned out that for every extra thirty minutes of driving, commuters had a 3 percent greater chance of being obese than their walking peers. And those who lived less than a half mile from stores were 7 percent less likely to become obese than their friends who had to drive to shop. The study also said that suburban white men typically weigh about ten pounds more than men who live in dense urban areas that feature shops and services within walking distance.

Food for Thought

"The more driving you do means you're going to weigh more—the more walking means you're going to weigh less."

Dr. Laurence Frank
Georgia Tech[6]

Increased TV Viewing and Computer Use

Most kids today grow up with television. Yet studies consistently show that the more they watch TV, the fatter they tend to be. With kids the "magic number" is around two hours a day. The Institute of Medicine recommends that parents limit their children's recreational TV, video game, and computer time to less than two hours a day.[7]

Anything over two hours a day and the tendency toward obesity rises almost in lockstep with the amount of TV watched (see Chapter 7, "From Boob Tube to Mean Screen").

Food for Thought

The more TV kids watch, the fatter they tend to be.

Reduced Safe Environments

Many parents don't let their children go outside and play as in days gone by, out of a genuine concern for their safety. With child abductions, drive-by shootings, gang activity, and drug use seemingly on the rise every year, Mom and Dad just don't want their sons and daughters out on the streets without adult supervision. So the kids stay inside, where they're less active . . . and they get heavier as a result.

Reduced Participation in Physical Education Classes and School Athletics

In these days of shrinking school budgets and increased pressure on students to pass standardized tests, many schools have eliminated physical education requirements. As a result, kids aren't burning off even the minimal calories that they did in earlier times. Even recess is getting cut out for many schoolkids.

Food for Thought

"Without any question, the No. 1 barrier to physical activity in schools is the misperception that time spent in PE and recess will undermine academic learning."

Charles Corbin
Arizona State University

At the same time, after-school athletics are shrinking in many places, again often due to budget shortfalls. In many districts students who do participate on sports teams have to pay for the privilege, which further diminishes participation. All of this is happening despite data that show the more a person exercises as a child, the more likely he or she is to exercise as an adult.

OTHER FACTORS TO CONSIDER

Beyond eating more and exercising less, many experts point to other factors that have contributed to the current crisis of childhood obesity. Consider three of the most important.

Obese and Overweight Parents

Study after study has shown that overweight parents tend to produce overweight kids. For the most part, this is *not* due to genetics, but to bad habits and poor lifestyles that parents model. In other words, overweight couch potatoes are, with rare exceptions, raised, not born.

And overweight kids do *not* tend to lose their unhealthful pounds, but rather carry them right into adulthood. We see this unfortunate phenomenon every day in our clinical practices; the kids who weigh the most almost invariably have obese parents, siblings, and relatives.

Family lifestyles and traditions play a much larger role in the problem of obesity than heredity does. Children are far more likely to do what's caught than what's taught. They'll do what they see their parents doing, rather than what the parents say they ought to do.

Food for Thought

Family lifestyles and traditions play a much larger role in the problem of obesity than heredity.

A Preference for Extra Pounds

While on a book tour a few weeks ago, Walt ran into a longtime friend. "You just look so good!" she exclaimed when she saw him.

Walt regrets that at the time his BMI was about 28 (which put him in the overweight category); he weighed more then than when he played rugby in college. Scott, his son, had just told him, "Dad, your support walls are sagging!" So he replied to his friend, "Oh, thanks, but I'm really not. I weigh too much."

"Oh, no, no, *no!*" his friend insisted. "Last time you were here, you did not look healthy."

When he last saw her, he was at a normal BMI. Like far too many in America, she saw an overweight person as a normal and healthy person.

Sherri's grandmother is the same way. She's always telling Sherri that she doesn't eat enough or weigh enough. And her mom always says that she brought the wrong baby home; Sherri's the only one in the family with a normal BMI.

Here's the truth: Some generations and cultures do not see obesity as a problem, but as a blessing. They see extra pounds as a sign of good health, not bad health. And they see a normal-weight child as an unhealthy child.

That's just one of the many reasons that the obesity crisis has reached such profound levels among certain ethnic groups—for example, Hispanics and African Americans. Jorge Cruz, the author of *Eight Minutes in the Morning,* has said, "We as Latinos have to have a wake up call. Food is not love. And we destroy our health if we don't change."[8]

Parents from generations and cultures like the ones just mentioned do not tend to see themselves or their children as overweight. They see the extra pounds not only as normal but as healthful. And this perception presents a huge obstacle to genuine health.

Physicians Ill Prepared to Tackle Childhood Obesity

The American Academy of Pediatrics has noted that most physicians who attended medical school more than twenty years ago received little training in nutrition, primarily because childhood obesity simply was not a big problem. Moreover, physicians aren't used to seeing adult diseases in kids. They haven't had to face it before, and many feel uneasy about addressing the problem.

Walt usually tells parents that they should not depend on their primary physician alone to deal with this problem. Yes, he or she can help to monitor blood pressure, blood sugar, BMI, etc., but if they want to overcome this threat, they'll need more than the help of their primary care physician. They'll need to pursue a team approach. And the child's physician and registered dietitian can work with the parent and child to help prevent or treat SuperSizing.

SUPERSIZE ME

SuperSize Me became a smash hit at the 2004 Sundance Film Festival by exposing fast-food mania in America. The producer decided to make himself a guinea pig and run an experiment, which he filmed. Under the supervision of three doctors, he started eating only items on the McDonald's menu, three times a day, every day for an entire month; and if an employee asked him to "supersize" anything, he did.

Viewers of the film had to stomach this man gorging himself on burgers, fries, and sugary soft drinks. Many expressed amazement at the damage he did to himself in only thirty days. His blood pressure and cholesterol level skyrocketed; he suffered liver damage; came down with headaches and depression; gained twenty-five pounds; reportedly lost his libido; and felt chest pains.

The film's producer—and its victim—was Morgan Spurlock, who has said, "I just hope the film can continue to inspire people as it has all around the world. Film [has] a great way of putting across a very serious message but in a way that people can stomach. It's not preachy; it's very palatable; it's a fun movie and so I hope people walk out of this film thinking about the choices they make in their lives."[9]

Unfortunately the damage Mr. Spurlock did to himself in his film is repeated in a stunning percentage of our children—and the consequences will be no less devastating.

So is that it? Are we done? Have we already eaten ourselves to death? Have we run out of both time and hope?

No, not quite yet. There's still time to turn this mess around and avoid the devastating consequences of allowing our kids to keep getting heavier. There is indeed still hope! And now we'd like to start showing you how to find it.

4

THERE'S STILL TIME

Do you remember the story of Sarah from Chapter 1? Although her story ended tragically, Sarah may have saved the life of her brother, Hershel. He'll live much longer because of a decision her parents made.

When Walt saw four-year-old Hershel the first time, it was for his first well-child checkup. He was happily sucking on a baby bottle filled with a cola, following the pattern of his older siblings. And, like them all, he wasn't just overweight—he was fat.

After Sarah died, however, her mother and father finally felt motivated to make some health-directed changes and came to see Walt. He could not have been happier for them, and they had really already begun, because the first step to reversing or preventing your kids from becoming SuperSized is to decide to do so.

However, Walt knew the entire family still had a long journey in front of them. He also knew that if he could give them some simple, doable steps, they would begin to see success early on, which would motivate them to make even more changes.

They started slow and kept their goals low. But they made progress! The family gradually changed its nutrition habits. The kids got involved in sports, and even the parents began to exercise. Five years later all of Sarah's siblings had a normal BMI. And while Mom and Dad were still overweight, they were no longer obese.

Walt had never felt worse than when Sarah died, and he never felt better than when he attended Hershel's high school graduation. Hershel was an attractive, intelligent, and healthy young man who, unlike his sister, had been given the opportunity for a long and robust life by a loving mom and dad who made the decision not to have SuperSized children and not to remain SuperSized themselves.

This story shows that despite the gathering storm clouds and the ominous rumble of thunder, we have much room for hope. In fact, we already have all the power we need to avert this crisis and turn things around in America. We have the ability to take control of our health and break the grip of obesity on ourselves and our families. We can choose to take decisive action to help our kids move from fat to fit.

Does that sound surprising to you, given the bleak picture we've painted so far? Make no mistake, we face a real and frightening crisis—but we can tackle the problem with all kinds of hope. We're sure of this because already we have seen many individuals, schools, and communities turn the corner. At the core of our hope lie many solid pieces of evidence. Let's take a look at a few of them.

INCREASING AWARENESS OF THE PROBLEM

Perhaps the best news is that more and more of us are becoming aware of the growing obesity epidemic. Everywhere you turn these days, talk of obesity seems to take center stage. It's become a hot topic, and that's good.

The way we look at it, the more of us who start grasping the problem, the greater the chance that it can be overcome in time. As public awareness grows, informed action has a better chance of following.

That goes for the physicians who care for our children as well. As knowledge of childhood obesity increases, a growing number of physicians will become aware, not only of what to look for but also of what to do once they spot a problem. They can then begin to play a key role in intervention and help us to get our kids back on the right track.

SMALL CHANGES BRING BIG RESULTS

Despite the enormity of the problem, even small changes in the way we live can make a huge difference in the quality of our children's health. By making small but significant changes now, we can set up our kids to enjoy many happy and productive years. Consider a few of the following changes in lifestyle:

- Encouraging increased physical activity early in life (ages four to eleven) can reduce the incidence of obesity and get kids started on health-promoting habits that will stay with them even into adulthood.
- Reducing caloric intake by even one hundred calories per day—one chocolate chip cookie—can prevent or begin to reverse unhealthy weight gain.
- Cutting down or eliminating soft drinks can result in significant weight reduction.
- Dining at home as a family can have a marked effect on reducing weight gain, as well as improving a family's physical, emotional, and relational health.
- Reducing or eliminating TV viewing and computer/video game time can result in significant weight reduction, lowering of cholesterol, and increased fitness.
- Refusing to eat meals in front of the TV can help avoid significant weight gain.
- Learning to cut portion sizes, feeding your children a healthy breakfast, and teaching them to choose healthy snacks have almost immediate effects.

None of these changes require family members to alter their lives completely. But putting into practice any one of them can result, over time, in enormous health benefits. Yes, there's reason for hope! And in subsequent chapters we'll talk in more detail about these and other small, easy, and effective steps you can take to begin.

REVERSE THE CONSEQUENCES

We know we can defeat the national crisis of childhood obesity and we also know that if we can get our kids healthy now, they'll avoid the serious physical problems that would plague them later as obese adults. Yes, some obese kids already suffer from many of the health challenges that once afflicted only obese adults; but a growing number of studies show that by reducing their weight and getting healthy, these same kids can *reverse* the health deficits caused by carrying around too many pounds as children.

- Modest weight reduction and daily exercise decrease high blood pressure, lipid abnormalities, and blood sugar levels.
- Increased physical activity can reduce the likelihood of developing diabetes and vascular disease.
- Dropping unhealthy pounds can reduce the chance of developing atherosclerosis (commonly referred to as hardening of the arteries, a condition where the arteries become narrow due to cholesterol deposits), and atherosclerosis in obese children improves as a result of exercise training.
- Lifestyle interventions can decrease the tendency to develop type 2 diabetes in adults; we have every reason to think that the same thing would hold true for kids.
- Females who intentionally reduced their weight enjoyed a 20 percent reduction in mortality, much of this from a decrease in obesity-related cancers. Mortality associated with diabetes decreased by 30 to 40 percent.

Food for Thought

By preventing obesity early in life, it appears that many cancers can be avoided.

Some people, like Hershel's mom and dad, find the motivation to take off or keep off unwanted pounds by remembering a loved one who fell victim to obesity.

Another patient of Walt's carefully preserved a picture of his grandma, a woman the size of the *Titanic* who had a great fondness for baking bread. He loved his grandma and he cherished that picture. Yet Walt can remember him saying, time and again, "I just don't want to be like her." He loved her, admired her, respected her—but he absolutely did not want to wind up morbidly obese, like her. That photo provided great motivation for him to keep trim.

We know of few motivators greater than the desire to avoid cancer, especially among women. Recent news reports claim that obese women increase their colon cancer risk fourfold. We've known for some time that obese women increase their breast cancer risk. Why expose our children to such risks if we don't have to?

The earlier we can catch these physical problems—and the earlier our kids can shed their extra pounds, begin physical activity, and improve their nutrition—the better chance we have at reversing the damage. Early detection and prevention are key. This means there is hope . . . as long as we act soon.

IT'S NEVER TOO EARLY TO START

It's never too early to start our children down the road to a healthy life. We can start even before they're born, even before they're conceived. How? By remembering that obese parents tend to have obese kids. Overweight parents have overweight infants, who grow up to be overweight teens and adults.

Remember, the older the overweight child is, the smaller the chance that he or she will become a healthy weight for life. The older a person gets, the greater the chance of remaining obese for life (usually a much shorter one). Early intervention is by far the most effective strategy for long-term success.

Parents, the time to prevent or reverse SuperSizing in our kids is always *now*. Don't wait until the problem gets worse. Don't wait until serious physical problems appear. If your child has an apparent obesity problem, start today to deal with it. Why? An average-sized adult may have 20 billion to 30 billion fat cells; a moderately obese adult, however, can have 60 billion to 100 billion fat cells; and a morbidly obese person in excess of 300 billion fat cells. Obese children can have *five times* more fat cells than children of normal weight!

Once formed, these fat cells can decrease in size, but they do not decrease in number. Other than during the first year of life, the most fat cells form during the growth spurt of adolescence. Therefore, it is no surprise that studies have shown that good nutrition, exercise, and sleep habits in childhood (and the early teen years) result in lower numbers of fat cells and a dramatic decrease in the risk of obesity.

Second, as we age, our metabolism slows down in response to a decrease in muscle mass and less physical activity. This means our bodies burn fewer calories, making it more difficult to reverse obesity—and it may also become more difficult to deal with the serious consequences of those extra pounds.

Today is the best day to start!

YOU'RE THE QUARTERBACK

Anytime Sherri has a chance to interact with the young physicians training in Florida Hospital's family residency program, she is reminded that most still haven't received a lot of training in nutrition. So what do they do when they meet someone who needs help in that area? They refer the patient to an expert. If your child needs detailed advice in the area of diet and nutrition, you need to go to an expert—a nutritionist or dietitian—in addition to working with your child's physician.

But remember that you, the parent, are your child's health care quarterback—not the physician, not the dietitian, not the teacher at school. You can draft that physician or dietitian as a coach or adviser, but you can neither blame your physician for your child's obesity nor depend on him or her to get you out of this hole. It's up to *you* to put together your team and call the shots when it comes to your child's health.

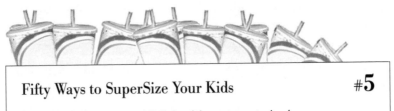

| Fifty Ways to SuperSize Your Kids | #5 |

Refuse to become your child's health care quarterback.

Several times parents have shown up in Sherri's office with their too-heavy kids, saying, "I'm concerned about my child's weight, but no one else seems to be. They don't think my child is overweight." Those parents know the child's family history—that the father's over-weight, as is Grandpa. So when they see a child putting on a few extra pounds, they take it upon themselves to act, rather than wait until a doctor or someone else says there's a problem. And that's just as it should be. That's exactly what a quarterback does!

If those around you have little interest in catching up with the latest information on childhood obesity, then you have the responsibility and the obligation to do so on your own. Find some supporters. And when it comes to your child's personal physician—who we believe should coach you—you also have to take charge. If your physician isn't coaching you well, find a different coach. That's your job.

"You mean I can fire my child's doctor?" You bet you can fire the doctor! He or she should be there to help you. You hire him or her to help *you* care for your child. You have the obligation to find someone who will empower, equip, and enable you to get the best health care possible for your kids.

Being your child's health care quarterback is a privilege and an opportunity. You may not have been calling the best plays, but you're still the leader. A recent AC Nielsen survey asked parents, "What is causing childhood obesity?" Do you know their overwhelming answer? "We are." Fast-food restaurants came in a distant second. It doesn't take a lot to convince parents that they need to do *something*; they just need some advice on *what* to do. They need some new plays.

As your coaches we want to provide you with ideas for some new plays to call. That's what this book is, your playbook. Have you ever seen a playbook? It's really thick, bursting with all kinds of plays. Of course, we don't expect you to learn them all or to do them all in one week. But you can start with *one* new one. If you're like most of us, you've been throwing Hail Mary passes for two years and have yet to score a touchdown. So why not learn how to do some solid and proven plays that any team can do. Try them out for a couple of games and then go from there.

Never forget that the responsibility for an overweight child rests with the parent. You can learn plays from all sorts of people, but *you* must call the plays. And in calling those plays, remember: It's not about weight loss alone.

- It is about more physical activity.
- It is about more sleep.
- It is about better eating.

Weight doesn't always come off as we'd like, but health-promoting habits can bring about positive change all by themselves, whether we see big weight loss or not. It's all about developing a healthy lifestyle, not just losing weight.

"I GIVE HIM ALL THE CREDIT"

Sixteen-year-old Tom came into our interview wearing a grin from ear to ear. He'd been losing weight ever since his freshman year in high school, when he stood about five feet eight inches tall and weighed 286 pounds (a morbidly obese BMI at 43.5). His doctor told him that he'd die of a heart attack by age forty-five if he didn't reach a healthier weight.

Tom says he started to "get big" around age ten; in fact, he weighed too much to play Pop Warner football. In ninth grade his golf coach told him he had to lose weight to get better at the sport and advised him to start walking more and to eat mustard rather than mayonnaise. He also started quizzing Tom about what he had eaten that day—and he was very good at sniffing out a lie. "If he ever saw me on a golf cart," Tom chuckled, "he'd have a fit."

Tom cut down on the size of his food portions and substituted mustard for mayonnaise. He cut down on the fries and eventually switched to baked potatoes. He also switched to diet soda. "That was the hardest," he said, not only because he likes regular soda but also because his friends gave him a hard time for choosing diet over regular.

Tom likes grapes and bananas and has always enjoyed salads, although now he's reduced the amount of dressing he puts on them. When he eats chips, he gets the baked variety, and he measures out his portion in a small cup. He manages the portions on his plate by keeping extra food away from the table instead of right in front of him.

For breakfast Tom usually has a Pop-Tart or maybe a Nutri-Grain bar. At school he looks for things like a turkey sub. When he hears a vending machine calling his name, he gets baked chips rather than the much fattier sour cream and onion option. He drinks a lot of water, maybe a case and a half of pint-sized bottles each week.

And he stays active. He plays golf and a lot of baseball and has worked as the student manager for the boys' basketball team at his school. In gym class he's taken courses in racquetball and weight training. He says he tries to stay active three days out of five. Even when he plays video games, he tries to opt for something active. "I just have to be moving," he says.

Tom tries hard to balance out his eating and activity levels. If he eats more than usual, he does something active to burn off the extra calories. And he eats less if he knows he's not going to be active. "I don't like to sit at home and be a couch potato," he declares.

His sleeping habits have also changed (see Chapter 6, "The Crucial Importance of R.E.S.T."). During school he hits the sheets about 10:30 P.M.; during the summer he goes to bed as late as 2 A.M., but then doesn't get up until late morning. He says he sleeps much better these days and doesn't feel nearly as tired as he used to.

All of these changes have paid off handsomely. Today Tom stands about five ten and weighs 238 pounds—a drop of almost fifty pounds (and a reduction in his BMI to a much better 34, which also reduces his risk of diabetes and premature heart disease). And he's still losing weight.

Recipe for Success

Mom and Dad: *You're* the key to preventing SuperSized Kids.

Tom credits some of his success to his mom and dad, his health care quarterbacks. Perhaps thinking of her own parents, who both suffered from diabetes, his mother joined Weight Watchers. Halfway through her program, Tom's dad joined her; eventually he lost fifty-two pounds. When Tom saw how well it was going for both of his parents, he started on his own weight reduction program. His parents didn't pressure him—he did it on his own—but his parents led the way! When his weight fluctuated a bit, he tried to stay positive. He saw his mom keeping at it, and that kept him going. He says he'd like to stay at 210 to 220 pounds.

"I give him all the credit," his dad said proudly several times during our interview. "I commend him. I think it's more of a way of life for him now."

The weight loss and healthier lifestyle have done wonders for Tom's confidence level. "It was like night and day," marvels his dad. Tom's endurance level has also shot way up. And his friends have noticed.

Homecoming, Tom says, "was a real eye-opener." He received "a ton" of compliments, and he believes the girls have started noticing him much more than they used to. He also likes to look at a photo of himself taken at the beach two years ago. "When I see it now," he said, "it makes me feel really good about how far I've come."

Does Tom have a message for others? He thinks about the question for a moment and then tells about a friend "who weighs 330 pounds of solid fat." This friend has a very large mother and really struggles with his weight. Some of Tom's other friends joke that the young man has three girlfriends: Aunt Jemima, Sara Lee, and Little Debbie. But Tom would like to tell his friend something else.

"Think of what could happen," Tom says. "Think of the positives— the whole Jared thing." Jared, you'll remember, became famous for his television commercials about losing weight by eating low-fat Subway sandwiches. Tom didn't follow Jared's regimen, but he does show us that our kids *can* turn things around—if we give them the right guidance and encouragement.

And there's great hope in that!

A BUFFET OF OPTIONS

"But I think it will just be too hard," you might say. "I'm not sure I can do it."

We don't think it's too hard to make the lifestyle changes that most books ask you to make; we think it's *impossible*. Because we take care of real people every day in our real-life practices, we want to encourage you, not make you pull out your hair. We want you to be a success and not a failure. We want to do everything we can to set you on a road of achievement and accomplishment—on the road to win!

In our prescription for your kids, we'll give you a menu, a smorgasbord, a buffet of options that are easily doable. We won't be asking you to do them all; pick just one at a time. Don't select the one *we* like; choose the one(s) *you* prefer, and then follow through. We know from experience that if you settle on one that you think your family can do, you're far more likely to follow through. And as you begin to see success with that one, it feels a whole lot easier to add a second one and then maybe a third one.

We don't want you or your kids to become yo-yo dieters. We want you to make the changes that you want to make, that will benefit your family's health, and that will have a multigenerational, positive impact on your whole clan. We want you to pick the strategies that fit your temperament; that fit your life stage; that fit your lifestyle. You wouldn't be reading this book if you didn't want to do *some*thing!

This is evidence-based, trustworthy information that can help you to deal with the serious problem of childhood obesity. There's good news here! There's great hope here!

Yes, we face a growing epidemic, but already we have effective ways of dealing with it. We'll learn more as the years go on, but right now we know of many things that really work that you can put into practice, starting today. And the quicker you start, the better for both you and your family.

There really is hope! To find it for yourself, turn the page and begin using a new playbook for your family's health.

PART TWO

Taking Kids from Fat to Fit

5

THE FAMILY BUSINESS

One night when the Larimore children were preteens, the family decided to stop speeding down the expressway of life long enough to share dinner. Walt always enjoyed mealtimes with his family because it gave everyone the opportunity to visit and catch up with each other. His wife, Barb, had laid down the law: The family would share as many meals together as possible. Period!

On this evening Scott, their youngest, made an observation that froze everyone in midchew.

"Dad," he began, "don't you think we're all getting a little bigger than we should?"

Barb blushed and Walt remembers his mouth dropping open. At that time in the Larimore family history, Scott was the one who most needed to lose some weight. Walt thought, *Isn't this the pot calling the kettle black?* But before he could say anything, Scott continued, "I think we could *all* stand to lose a bit of weight."

Walt looked over at Barb. She smiled and then looked at Scott, once more busy with his plate. "Scott, I think you've brought up something important for us to talk about," she said. Then she turned to Kate. "What do you think, honey?"

Kate shrugged her teenage shoulders.

Walt looked down at his midriff, which had begun to show the middle-age sag so common in men his age.

"Well," continued Barb, "let's figure out what we need to do as a family. What do you all say?"

That night they began an important discussion about what they could do *as a family* about hurtling down the dangerous road of SuperSizing. They knew they needed to get off that road. They knew that their family lifestyle, left uncorrected, could become a recipe for disaster. So they decided to change, one step at a time, starting that night.

The Larimores knew that they weren't exercising enough, that they ate more often than they should at fast-food restaurants, and that their diets contained an unhealthy amount of sugar and saturated fat. Moreover, they had stopped the habit of eating together as a family and had begun eating some meals in front of the television. They knew they needed to improve.

As a first step they chose as a family to keep a daily diary of what each family member ate. At the end of one month they had another family discussion. They discovered they had eaten only nine dinners together. All of them had often skipped breakfast and had consumed a surprisingly high number of soft drinks and an unexpectedly large amount of snack food. Their meeting ended with a decision to do some fact-finding.

During the next two months they read books on improving family nutrition. Barb purchased a couple of cookbooks with health-oriented recipes, and each of them picked recipes he or she wanted to try. They learned the difference between "good" and "bad" fats, carbohydrates, and proteins. They learned about how a child's nutritional needs differ from those of adults. They learned how to select snacks low in saturated fats, trans fats, and sugars.

As we've mentioned frequently, nutritional habits are not as easily taught as they are caught. Barb and Walt came to the sobering realization that they needed to demonstrate good nutrition before their children would practice it. They came to understand the necessity of good exercise and activity habits for their children, which meant they needed to do those activities with them.

Armed with facts and ideas, they came prepared to make some key decisions at their next family meeting. Those decisions continue to impact their family's health. As a result:

- They feel better.
- They have more energy.
- They sleep better.
- They have lost weight and kept it off.

Food for Thought

Six big facts the Larimores learned:

1. Some fats *are good*.
2. Some fats are awful.
3. Kids over two years old need nonfat milk and dairy products.
4. Nutrition labels help parents pick foods low in sugar, salt, and bad fat.
5. Chocolate is not a food group—but is okay once in a while.
6. Sodas can be dangerous. Water gives life.

What kept Barb and Walt from making these changes years before? Their experience dovetailed with one national survey that indicated that while 70 percent of parents want good nutrition and eating habits for their children, only 40 percent thought they had succeeded.[1] The gulf between desire and success will continue to exist as long as parents neglect to match their words with their actions. Most parents fail to teach good eating habits to their kids, not because they lack information, but because they don't practice good habits themselves. And if you don't model it, you're not going to succeed in teaching it.

Whether you're a mom, a dad, a grandparent raising your grandkids, or a legal guardian of children, *you* set the tone in your home. The physical, emotional, relational, and spiritual environment you create goes a very long way toward setting up your kids for a long and successful life.[2]

WHOSE PROBLEM IS IT?

America's kids will not slim down until America's families—both adults and children—start living markedly healthier lifestyles. That's the unvarnished truth from medical experts across the nation.

One group of experts, for example, surveyed all of the recent studies on childhood obesity and concluded, "All risk factors for the development of childhood overweight have their initial beginnings in the family of origin." The group also declared, "Therefore, an overweight child cannot be effectively treated in isolation of the family."[3]

In days gone by, efforts to reduce childhood obesity focused largely on the behavior of the child and placed the burden of change squarely on the shoulders of that child. And you know what? It didn't work. That's why the most up-to-date studies agree that efforts that "encourage weight loss among children *and their parents* have greater long-term success rates than programs focusing solely on child weight reduction" (italics added).[4]

A high percentage of parents with overweight children who come in to see Sherri for help and advice on nutrition consider the visit, not a family concern, but something that affects only the obese child. They tend to sit silently in the corner while expecting the child to interact with Sherri—and some of these kids are only six and seven years old! When the child starts wondering aloud why his sister can eat potato chips, but he can't, Mom and Dad continue to sit there quiet as mice. And when Sherri glances toward the adults and suggests a few things that might help the child to lose weight, nine times out of ten the parents look at the child and say, "Listen to her. She's talking to *you*." Almost never do they step in to say, "Okay, we'll go grocery shopping together and make our food choices as a family." Many parents totally remove themselves from the process, no matter what the age of the child.

Now, if the child were a seventeen- or eighteen-year-old, that would be one thing; they're old enough to go to the grocery store alone and make better food choices on their own. But a six-year-old?

He or she is totally at the mercy of the parent regarding what is available to eat. However, too frequently the parents have completely stepped back from the issue; they believe it's not *their* problem, but the *child's* problem. And an attitude like that almost guarantees that the child will never reach a healthy weight.

Sad to say, no parent has yet said to Sherri, "We're concerned with Johnny's weight, and the whole family is committed to doing something about it." Very rarely will the parent even say, "I'm committed to helping him." Too often Mom or Dad brings in the child and expects Sherri to impart some easy, bright ideas to fix the problem. These days, when Sherri gets silent parents who want to do nothing but sit and listen, she tries to pull them to the table and teach them how to become their child's health care quarterback.

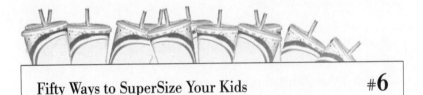

Fifty Ways to SuperSize Your Kids   #6

Consider your kid's SuperSize status *their* problem and not a *family* problem.

As in Sherri's experience, and in Walt's more than twenty years as a family physician, only a few families looked at this as a family problem. The parents of one such family were overweight but not obese. Their obese son, John, suffered from asthma and complained of knee pain. Both of their other two children suffered from poor health; one wrestled with a depressive disorder.

Like most of his patients, the mother brought in John so Walt could "fix his problem." John was, after all, the "patient." But Walt had to get the mom to see that this problem was not just John's, but the whole family's.

"I have some good news and some better news!" Walt announced. "The good news is that this is all changeable. I want to give you hope and help. Okay?"

The mom nodded. "However," Walt continued, "the even better news is that, for Johnny to get better, it's not only Johnny who's got to change, but the whole family."

The mom looked shocked at first. Then Walt could see her mental wheels turning. Finally she nodded, and a look of determination settled on her face. Walt recommended she arrange a *family* conference with a dietitian—and she did.

That week she and John's father met with a registered dietitian who began the process of teaching options for improving the health of *every* family member, including John. Over the next six months, by implementing one small step at a time, the family made wholesale changes to their nutrition:

- More home-cooked meals
- More family dining
- Less TV and no eating in front of the TV
- Less fast food on the run
- Big reductions in sweets and sugary foods
- Walking as a family before supper, which increases metabolism and in a weird sort of way made them less hungry

Within two years the entire family had slimmed down. John looked great, his knees stopped bothering him, bullies no longer harassed and ridiculed him at school, and his breathing problems disappeared. When his sister's depressive disorder also stabilized, this family became one of the real success stories of Walt's practice.

When parents accept their role as health quarterbacks and take charge of their children's fitness, kids start shedding pounds like an animal's winter coat on a warm spring day.

Jean Wiecha, a senior research scientist at the Harvard School of Public Health, points out the crucial place of parental involvement:

"Parents can create an environment in the home that encourages good health by having an assortment of healthy foods around, by making sure that there are limits set on television, and having meals as a family in the evening."[5]

Changing long-held family eating habits requires not only parental involvement but parental discipline. Focus on the Family's psychologist-in-residence, Dr. Bill Maier, says that busy parents often feel loath to restrict what their children eat because they feel guilty for working so much. Taking the family out for fast food during the week and letting the kids order a supersized meal is viewed by these parents as a "treat."

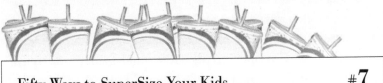

Fifty Ways to SuperSize Your Kids   #7

Fail to teach your kids good eating habits, especially when they are young.

Keep in mind, too, that young children learn good habits much more readily than do older kids or teens. If you want to make a life-long impact on your child's nutritional habits and spare him or her countless diseases for many years to come, you can't do better than to start teaching and modeling good habits before that youngster reaches five years of age.

Here's the truth: The whole family needs to get involved. Not only do we need Junior and Missy to lose those dangerous extra pounds, we need Mommy and Daddy to get fit and unfat as well. It's really about involving the whole family in creating a lifestyle of nutritious eating, good physical habits, and total family wellness.

THE NUMBER ONE INFLUENCER

"Now, wait a minute," you might be saying. "Do you expect me to believe that I have the most influence over what and how my kids eat? What about peers? What about sports superstars and Hollywood types? What about TV and all those advertisements? Don't those affect my kids more than me?"

Not according to virtually all experts and recent studies. If you're a parent who wants to know the number one influencer on your kids in regard to eating and exercise, you need look nowhere else but in the mirror.

Parents really do have the most impact over what their kids eat—more than sports stars, famous celebrities, or other kids, according to Cynthia Sass, R.D., a nutritionist and a spokeswoman for the American Dietetic Association. "Parents have a fundamental role to teach their child healthy habits at home," she said. "If the family as a whole is trying to consume more vegetables, it's going to impact how small children eat."[6]

Food for Thought

Parents of SuperSized Kids are often overweight or obese themselves.

We parents tend to get this flip-flopped. And yet we really do tend to have far more influence over what and how our kids eat and exercise than does anyone else.

One study has demonstrated "the long-term (ten-year) effectiveness of a combined parent-child intervention program" by showing that obese children placed in a family-based weight reduction program lost more weight and consumed more healthful food than children treated with a more conventional approach that expected the kids to police themselves.[7] "Parents need to be the main agents of change," concludes the study. "The home and family environments are major factors affecting the child's knowledge, beliefs, attitudes, and practice regarding food and eating habits. Moreover, directing children to diet and to slim down may predispose the obese child to eating disorders."[8]

Translation: Nobody has more of an influence on what and how your children eat and exercise than you do, Mom and Dad. And if you leave weight issues to your kids to solve, chances are they'll not only stay fat, they'll also be at higher risk for developing dangerous medical conditions.

Food for Thought

As a parent you can model choices and behavior that will favorably impact your child's health. As his or her health care quarterback your behavior is the most powerful play you have!

THEY LEARN BEST BY EXAMPLE

Sherri and her husband are very good friends with another couple who have a thirteen-year-old son. That boy refuses to touch mushrooms. And do you know why? His father hates them. The boy's dislike of mushrooms seems to have nothing to do with his not liking the taste or texture of a mushroom; he says he's never even tried one. He's just heard his dad say all his life how terrible mushrooms are. So this young man won't go anywhere near them. Even though the father has tried to be careful about saying he doesn't like mushrooms, it seems his actions have spoken louder than his words.

Would you believe that this family's experience is validated by rigorous scientific studies? Two medical researchers recently concluded, "It is probable that children will want to eat, and through repeated exposure, learn to like foods that they see their parents eating."[9]

Texas Children's Hospital agrees. Experts there say, "Children learn by example. Eat a variety of healthful food and be physically active every day so that your children will learn healthful habits."[10] Yet another pair of experts claims, "Studies show that . . . attitudes about food and eating are learned and reinforced within the home."[11]

But why should this surprise anyone? Parents provide children with their first models of many activities, including eating and exercise behavior. Therefore, "Parents who overeat, eat excessively fast, or ignore their internal satiety [feeling full] clues provide a poor example for their children. It is up to them to present a healthy eating style in the home and external social environment, to model healthy selection and consumption of foods, and to engage in regular physical activity."[12]

Recipe for Success

You are the most influential model your kids have.

You are the most influential model your kids have. Not Jimmy down the street. Not Madonna on the tube. Not King James on the court. *You*. Kids learn best by example, and whether you like it or not, *your* example influences your kids' eating and exercise behavior more than that of anyone else.

OBESE PARENTS RAISE OBESE KIDS

It's especially important to recognize the crucial role you play as the prime example for your children regarding weight issues, for the simple but profound reason that obese parents tend to raise obese kids. We've said it before, but it bears repeating: Obese parents tend to raise obese kids.

One study found that "the risk of adult obesity was greater in both obese and non-obese children if at least one parent was overweight."[13] The journal *Pediatrics* reported that "for young children, if one parent is obese, the odds ratio is approximately 3 for obesity in adulthood, but if both parents are obese, the odds ratio increases to more than 10. Before three years of age, parental obesity is a stronger predictor of obesity in adulthood than the child's weight status."[14]

Don't miss the startling conclusion here: If one parent is obese, his or her children are three times more likely to become obese than a child without an obese parent. But if that child has two parents considered obese, his or her chance of becoming an obese adult rises to *ten times* that of a child with parents of normal weight. That's staggering! Why would any of us want to expose our kids to such terrible odds?

DIFFERING PERCEPTIONS

Sometimes we unknowingly subject our children to unacceptable health risks because we simply don't perceive childhood obesity as a threat. This seems especially true of certain demographic groups.

Maybe a household includes several members of an extended family. Mom and Dad might recognize the terrible danger of carrying around too many extra pounds, but maybe Grandpa or Grandma does not. Probably they grew up with a radically different mind-set and so feel determined to bring home the Twinkies and the Oreos. And, in fact, one group of researchers says that "children believe that grandparents and elderly aunts give them what they want despite parental disapproval. Parents also indicated that grandmothers, when they perceive that their grandchildren are thin, may conclude that the mothers are inadequately feeding the children."[15]

Cultural differences regarding food and weight can also add to the problem. Mothers from the South Pacific islands of Micronesia, for example, perceive thinness to be a result of illness and therefore do not mind those extra pounds on their kids.[16]

But we don't have to wander from the shores of America to find such differences. In one study of "significantly obese African-American children, many parents did not perceive their children as very over-weight, nor did they feel that weight was a health problem for their child . . . many African-American parents do not perceive morbid obesity as a pediatric-health concern."[17]

As we have already seen, however, childhood obesity *is* a national health concern, one that needs to be addressed immediately. And how can it best be addressed? The best answer: in a total family context that involves the whole clan. No other remedy works anywhere near as effectively.

ACCEPT THEM AND ENCOURAGE THEM

Overweight children probably know better than anyone else that they have a weight problem; for that reason they need the support, accept-ance, and encouragement of parents.

Rather than scolding a child for being obese, tell your child he or she is loved, special, and important. Children's feelings about them-selves are largely based upon their parents' attitude toward them. Children are more likely to accept themselves when their parents accept them. Do they need to change their behavior to reduce their weight? Certainly. But look for positive ways to enhance their self-esteem and so motivate them to change. Here's the key: Love your children regardless. Love them "in spite of." Love them unconditionally.

Children cannot become as healthy as possible without parental affirmation and approval. Boys want to know, from their parents, "Do I have what it takes? Am I becoming a man in your eyes?" Girls want to know, "Am I lovely? Am I precious? Am I worthy of pursuit?" Quite simply your children need you to be their best cheerleader. You get to be not only their health care quarterback but their cheerleader, too. What a deal!

Recipe for Success

SuperSized Kids cannot win the battle over obesity without the continual coaching and cheering of their parents.

Think about it: If you're not cheering on your children, who is? They need your "atta boy" and "way to go" and "I'm so proud of you," more than you know. Too many parents major in critique and forget to cheer. And when obesity assaults a child's self-concept and self-worth, he or she needs the parents' affirmation even more.

If someone tells us, "You should be doing this," but has rarely bothered to spend much quality time with us or to really get to know us, we're less likely to listen—even if what he or she says is true. But if someone really cares about us and takes the time to understand us and makes it known that he or she really likes us for who we are, then suddenly we become much more open to listening.

In the same way, unless you build a positive relationship with your children, they're not likely to listen to what you have to say regarding their food and exercise choices. If an overweight child feels your constant disapproval or demands, you'll only worsen his or her already damaged self-esteem. And that child won't feel any desire to do anything about the extra weight. *I'm worthless anyway,* he or she is likely to think, *so why even try?* Many studies show that positive feedback works much more effectively to encourage needed change than does negative input.

So listen to your children's concerns about their weight. Let them know that you care. And whatever you do, make it a habit to tell your child that he or she is loved, is special, and is important to you.

Weight control begins in the mind—and you, more than anyone, have the ability to affect what goes on up there.

WHERE DO I START?

Maybe this idea of weight control as a family affair is new to you. If so, where do you start to make needed changes? What's the best way to begin?

Know Your Current Habits

When a family asks Sherri to help them get started down the right track, the first thing she does is find out what's currently happening under their roof.

"Okay," she'll say, "tell me what a typical day for you is like. When do you get up? What do you eat for breakfast? Do you eat together? What kind of food do you stock? What kind of exercise does every member of the family enjoy? When do you go to bed? What kind of television habits do you have?"

Of course, Sherri knows that when someone tells her about their eating and exercising habits, they're usually giving her only about 75 percent of the truth. It seems to be human nature to underestimate how much we eat and overestimate how much we move. If they tell her they're having only one soda a day, for example, usually it's a safe bet that they're actually having two or three. Still, it's always best to try to discover what routines already exist within a family and then help them brainstorm a few things that they are willing to change or to start doing.

You can do the same thing on your own. As of this moment, what kind of eating habits does your family have? How much do you exercise? It doesn't hurt to monitor your family's habits for a couple of weeks; use a notebook to write down exactly what happens under your roof. You might think that you guzzle only one soda a day— but keeping a journal or diary of your actual experience might open your eyes.

It's a great place to start. Make sure you know your *real* starting place!

Eat Together

Many recent studies insist that eating together as a family has substantial effects on the control of obesity. A Harvard Medical School study of sixteen thousand children found that those who ate dinner more often with their parents ate more nutritious food and fewer calories.[18] Why?

First, the quantity and quality of food are easier to control when the family eats together. "Absence of family meals is associated with lower fruit and vegetable consumption as well as consumption of more fried food and carbonated beverages," said one medical journal.[19]

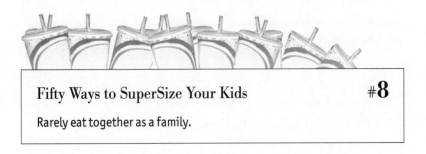

Fifty Ways to SuperSize Your Kids   #**8**

Rarely eat together as a family.

Second, eating together has positive effects on human emotions. One study concluded that quality family time is linked to good mental health in kids. "Sharing daily meals is a unifying ritual that promotes adolescent mental health," the study concluded.[20] A study published in the American Psychological Society newsletter found that teenagers who ate with their families five times or more a week were less likely to do drugs or be depressed, were more motivated at school, and had better peer relationships. And a survey of National Merit scholars from the past twenty years found that, without exception, these students came from families who ate together three or more nights a week.[21] Spending quality mealtimes together contributes to a child's mental and emotional health.

So what stops us from eating together as a family? Two of the most

> ### Recipe for Success
>
> Family mealtimes can build a child's mental and emotional health.

common causes are parents working late and children involved in extracurricular activities; it may be 8 P.M. or later before everyone gets home. Still, it's worth it to insist on family eating times, despite whatever obstacles stand in our way. It's certainly better to make health-promoting changes now than to suffer great regret a few years down the line.

One of our medical colleagues at Florida Hospital admits, "When my kids grew up, I was never there; they never really knew their daddy. We never ate meals together because I was never home. Daddy was always at the hospital, working."

> ### *Food for Thought*
>
> The family meal may be a lost art, but it's well worth recovering.

The family meal may be a lost art, but it's well worth recovering. We cannot urge you strongly enough to plan healthful meals and eat together as a family. Planning the week's meals can help save you time and money, while sitting together at mealtimes helps children learn to enjoy a variety of nutritious foods.

We have one big word of caution here. While it is perhaps parental nature to try to dictate to a child what and how much he or she should eat, it is now known that parents who attempt to overcontrol their children's eating actually add to the problem of obesity.[22] Don't forbid a food. If you tell a child she or he can never have a food, that food becomes all the more desirable.[23] One 2002 study found that young girls with mothers who restricted their food choices tended to snack excessively and eat even when they weren't hungry.[24] Most foods, when consumed in moderation, can be part of a generally healthful diet. By allowing the occasional consumption of foods you consider "junk," they become no big deal. In general, parents should be responsible for offering healthful foods, structured meals, and occasional snacks, while children should decide how much they eat.

One pair of experts writes that "by allowing children to make decisions about what and how much to eat, parents empower children to self-regulate their eating."[25] And in an article in *Time* magazine, Shannon Brownlee wrote:

> There's much that parents can do to influence the way their children eat and to lower the chances they will end up obese. Young children are keenly attuned to how many calories they need to grow and maintain a normal weight; they know when they are hungry and when they are full. But most kids quit listening to those internal cues by the time they reach school age. The reason? Parents, says Leann Birch, a psychologist at Penn State University. "There are things parents do with the best of intentions that turn out to be counterproductive," she says. A familiar example: insisting that children clean their plate, a rule that can teach kids to eat when they are not hungry.[26]

When it comes to family eating, the National Institutes of Health offers a good summary: "Involve the whole family in building healthy eating habits. It benefits everyone and does not single out the child who is overweight."[27]

Grocery-Shop Together

As much as possible, go grocery shopping together as a family. You can have all the best-laid plans in the world, but if you bring home junk food, you'll be setting up your family for dietary failure.

First, make a list of what you need. Most of the "impulse" buys we make tend to add fuel to the fire of childhood obesity. Begin the discipline of never letting your children talk you into buying anything not on the shopping list.

Second, don't go shopping on an empty stomach. Everything looks good when your stomach is growling.

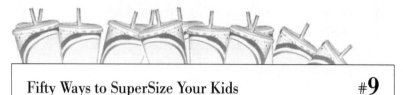

Fifty Ways to SuperSize Your Kids   #9

Make impulsive decisions (or let your kids talk you into impulsive decisions) while grocery-shopping.

Third, stick to the perimeter of the store; don't spend much time in the middle aisles. The most healthy food choices—like fruits and vegetables and dairy products—are usually arranged on the outside aisles, while the inside shelves generally get stocked with empty-calorie foods.

Fourth, skip buying soft drinks and high-fat/high-calorie snack foods like chips, cookies, and candy. If children do not see these foods at home, they will be less likely to ask for them and you will not have to say no. Instead, choose healthy snack foods (see Chapter 10, "Gearing Up for Healthy Family Meals"). Remember, if you fill your pantry with fatty snacks and sweet drinks, you're going to have to say no a lot—and that can make forbidden foods seem all the more desirable.

Exercise Together

The family that exercises together gets healthy together.

We know of one family that plays a game called Freeze Tag. They go outside in the fresh air two or three nights a week to play. The kid who is "it" must run around to catch and touch the other players to make them freeze, until they're all standing still. The family made this outdoor game such fun that now the kids beg to play it. It's a game that keeps you running, so you get great exercise, but it doesn't *feel* like exercise because you're playing the game as a family.

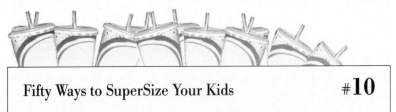

Fifty Ways to SuperSize Your Kids	#10
Don't involve your entire family in fun physical activity.	

It's important to make family activities fun, because you won't stick with them if they're not. Not far from metropolitan Orlando and Walt Disney World is something called the West Orange Trail, a former railroad track that has become a paved exercise path. It extends about nineteen miles on the north side of town. Eventually the trail will form part of a two-hundred-mile regional trail encircling Orlando, called the Central Florida Loop. It's wonderful to drive by the trail and see families on bikes or Rollerblades or walking together, having a great time. In response to the obesity epidemic many communities around the country are creating similar kinds of trails, parks, and outdoor recreation facilities for families and individuals. Check with your parks and recreation services to find out what's available in your area.

For those who like to run, many communities hold 5K and 10K runs, often accompanied by special kid runs of much shorter length. When kids see Mom or Dad training to run in a 5K or 10K, they often want to participate.

On our Web site, www.SuperSizedKids.com, we'll connect you with some resources that help kids to think of fun ways to become active. One site uses words like "bounce" and "jump" and other action verbs, which imply movement. The site sponsors little contests that encourage kids to get active. Parents, take note: Could you sponsor a mini fitness challenge of your own? You could set some exercise goals and tell the kids, "You get a certain number of points for each of these activities. When you get so many points, you can redeem them to buy a CD or toy." Kids definitely respond to rewards like this. (Remember that a hot fudge sundae is *not* an appropriate reward!)

Many health clubs offer not just family memberships but special programs for the kids. So while the parents work out in their part of the club, the kids can run around doing other active things, playing hopscotch or jump rope or kickball or basketball with small hoops or climbing a rock wall.

When you think family exercise, you have to look at the whole. If Dad is on the computer for five hours every night, it's going to be hard for the child to understand why he or she gets to sit in front of the glowing screen for only an hour each night. If a parent is always moaning and groaning because "I have to go work out," such an attitude rubs off on the kids.

The National Institutes of Health recommends, "Be active together as a family. Assign active chores such as making the beds, washing the car, or vacuuming. Plan active outings such as a trip to the zoo or a walk through a local park. Kids need a total of about sixty minutes of physical activity a day, but this does not have to be all at one time. Ten- or even five-minute bouts of activity throughout the day are just as good."[28]

Believe Together

Would it surprise you to learn that "trust in God" contributes to family health? More than sixteen hundred studies have shown that spiritual health is positively associated with physical, emotional, and relational health.[29]

Still, many people of faith also struggle with their weight.[30] Therefore, many faith communities have begun weight-loss programs. Many Christian houses of worship offer physical activities for their congregations and youth groups, everything from sports teams to game nights to camping trips, all of which encourage physical activity. Jewish and Muslim writers, too, are beginning to address religion and weight gain.[31]

Our Web site, www.SuperSizedKids.com, has a list of some currently available faith-based weight-loss programs around the country.

Furthermore, studies have shown that individuals who regularly attend a house of worship and who have a strong faith tend to have a better support group around them and therefore have less incidence of depression and mental anxiety. Because of this, they may be less susceptible to various kinds of emotional eating. In addition, strong social support has been shown to be helpful in adults who choose to improve their nutrition and lose weight.

Find Balance Together

As in most things, we must find balance in life. It doesn't necessarily follow that if sixty minutes of exercise a day is good, then five hours is even better. It's good for kids to get active and moving, but some families allow their children to get involved in far too many activities. Balance is the key.

The wife of a friend of ours teaches piano. She's had to have this discussion about balance more than once with parents of prospective students. They'll tell her that little Bobbie Sue is playing soccer and playing in the band and that she has about four other things going— and now she wants to take piano. And Lisa says, "You know, I don't think she does."

Many of us feel as though the more we do, the more meaning we bring to our lives. We think we'll feel better about ourselves when we can say, "Look at me, I'm so busy; that means my life has meaning." But it's most definitely *not* good for your health.

Consider just one common downside to the unbalanced life. You keep such a hectic schedule that you have only ten minutes to inhale your meal before you must be off to your next activity. Something has to give somewhere, so you hit the drive-through at a local fast-food place instead of going home and sitting down to a balanced meal. And before you know it, you get on the scale and the numbers have jumped ten notches.

That's not healthy. Not for you and not for your kids. Balance may not be easy to find, but it's worth searching for. And your scale will thank you.

THE NUMBER ONE DIET SABOTEURS

Who's most to blame when you or your child starts putting on those extra, unwanted pounds? The truth is, the number one diet saboteur is usually family and close friends.

Colleen Pierre of Johns Hopkins University says, "I've seen it happen so many times to my weight loss patients that when they come in and confess they fell off the wagon, I'm ready with my ritual response: 'Who did this to you?' They're always shocked to think that someone else may have had a hand in their weight loss failure. Diet saboteurs. They're everywhere."[32]

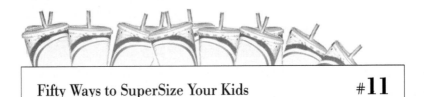

Fifty Ways to SuperSize Your Kids   #11

Let family or friends become diet saboteurs for your kids.

And how do they sabotage our diet? They give us cookies or offer us a candy bar or insist we have a second helping, just when we're getting on the right track. Often they don't realize what they're doing. Sometimes they do it because they feel guilty that whereas *we* seem to be losing weight, they're not. Or maybe they just don't understand; since they don't have a weight problem, they don't realize we can't go back to bad old habits just because we (or our kids) lost a few pounds. Others just miss "the old us."

Whatever the reasons, don't let the diet saboteurs keep you or your family from gaining control over your weight. They may be friends; they may be family; but don't let them derail your efforts to reach and maintain a healthy weight for every member of your family. Sabotage the saboteurs and *keep your family healthy*!

THE BEST ROUTE TO HEALTH

The leadership and good example of parents and guardians really do provide the best route to curing the top health crisis facing the American family. With the cost of obesity in America at a staggering $99.2 billion annually (and rising), we have our work cut out for us.[33]

Since childhood obesity afflicts more than Americans, experts from outside the United States are working on how best to combat it. Claudio Colistra, head of the Rome Federation of Pediatricians, has helped to launch a program to educate Italian parents and schools about good eating habits and the need for physical activity. "It all starts with the family," he said. "We have lost the habit of sitting down together, the whole family, and eating. We eat outside of the home now, we eat fast food, the mother works, snacks come packaged. Our task is to make parents reflect, and return to the old Italian culture."[34]

Food for Thought

"We have lost the habit of sitting down together, the whole family, and eating."

Dr. Claudio Colistra
Rome Federation of Pediatricians

Most Americans have no "old Italian culture" to return to, but we can learn from that culture and others like it about the necessity of tackling childhood obesity by using a total family approach.

Without question, childhood obesity presents an enormous challenge to the health of America and its kids. But when we meet that challenge as families, united and together, we really can win.

And you know what? We have no other choice.

SIMPLE STEPS THAT WORK

Remember that tackling your child's obesity is a family affair. Here are a few things you can do to get started together:

- Get to know your child's current eating habits. Uncover your child's perception of what is healthy eating and use the opportunity to correct any misconceptions.
- Remember, children are more likely to eat a food if they observe someone they respect enjoying that food. Let your kids watch and learn from your own good eating habits.
- Don't restrict how much your child is allowed to eat, or insist that your children clean their plates. Left to themselves, children are pretty good about eating just what they need.
- Encourage your children, when they are old enough, to serve themselves.
- Shop for food as a family. Make a list before going to the grocery store and stick to it. And don't fill your kitchen cupboards and refrigerator with unhealthy foods and soft drinks to tempt you and your kids.
- Sit down for dinner together as much as possible. Children eat better when Mom (or Dad) cooks and serves the food. Left to their own devices, most children would subsist on a diet of unhealthy processed food.
- Prepare meals together. Kids involved in the cooking are more likely to eat the results.
- Leave the television off during meals. The TV is a strong competitor for everyone's attention and keeps you from interacting

with one another. So keep it off during mealtime and never eat in front of it.

■ Let the phone ring. They're usually telemarketers, anyway. Let the answering machine pick up any messages.

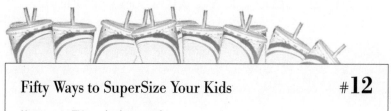

Fifty Ways to SuperSize Your Kids #12

Keep your TV on during meals.

6

THE CRUCIAL IMPORTANCE OF R.E.S.T.

When Walt's son, Scott, turned fifteen, the boy asked his parents if he could have a television in his bedroom. He even offered to pay for it.

Walt told Scott he would discuss his plea with his mom and get back to him. Since he did not know as much about the dangers of TV watching as he does now (and as we'll discuss in detail in the next chapter), he unwisely discounted Barb's feelings when she voiced her concerns. Barb is not only more intuitive than Walt; she is also a trained educator. Walt should have listened.

They discussed the potential positives and negatives, and she eventually gave in to Walt's point of view. So Walt told Scott he could get a TV as long as he bought it with his own money. Walt considered it a good lesson for him.

What a mistake! That TV attracted Scott like a vulture to a rotting carcass. The thing *sucked* him into his bedroom about fifteen seconds after he finished dinner, and no one saw him again until the next morning. Who knows what he watched? What a bad parenting move! Walt now says he should have listened to Barb.

So why are we telling you this story in a book on childhood obesity? The answer, we suspect, will surprise you.

With a TV in his bedroom Scott succumbed more times than not to the temptation to catch late-night shows on school nights. This cut into his sleep time and made him a lot more tired in the morning. Because he felt more tired, he began to exercise less in the afternoons, instead taking naps to catch up on his sleep. His morning fatigue led him to sleep later than he should, so instead of eating a healthful breakfast at home, he stopped at a fast-food restaurant on the way to school and gobbled down the food as he drove to class. As a result, his BMI began to shoot up.

What drove Scott's weight gain? Although a number of culprits could be identified, Walt never suspected back then that his son's lack of sleep and rest was one of them.

And we'll bet that what we're about to discuss will shock you, too.

ARE WE MISSING THE POINT?

Quick, now: What's the best diet for losing weight and getting healthy? Atkins? Weight Watchers? South Beach? Grapefruit? Salads only?

With questions like that, we might just be missing the point.

"We're in the middle of a diet debate over fats or carbohydrates [for optimal weight loss]," said Pam Smith, a registered dietitian and sports consultant based in Orlando, "but the part rest plays is missed in the debate."[1]

With all the media attention that this or that diet plan attracts, most people have no idea just how strong the link between sleep loss and weight gain is. An increasing number of studies are suggesting that the less sleep someone gets, the more likely he or she is to put on unwanted pounds. While scientists don't yet know the exact connection between the two, the link seems undeniable. And the few published studies that focus on the connection between sleep loss and weight gain in children ought to slap us wide awake.

The most comprehensive study to date looked at more than eight thousand Japanese children aged six to seven years. It found a "significant" connection between late bedtime or short sleeping hours and childhood obesity—that is, the fewer hours of sleep a child got, the more likely he or she was to be overweight or obese.[2]

Food for Thought

The less a child sleeps, the more likely he or she is to be SuperSized!

A second study focused on nearly seven thousand German children aged five to six. It found that the less these children slept, the more likely they were to be overweight or obese. Overweight children and those with excessive body fat also reported getting fewer hours of sleep than children of normal weight.[3]

In the United States, a survey of 1,473 randomly selected households conducted in 2004 found that children, from infants to fifth graders, are getting far less sleep than they need—a shortfall of one to two hours every night.[4]

Teens appear to follow a similar pattern. Researchers at the University of Texas Health Science Center in Houston discovered that obese adolescents slept significantly fewer hours than those of normal weight.[5] The Sleep Disorders Center at Henry Ford Hospital in Detroit interviewed more than a thousand teens and found that a third of them reported occasional sleep problems, while a whopping 94 percent of that group said they had had trouble sleeping at least twice a week for a month or longer during the previous year. Almost 20 percent of teens thirteen to sixteen years of age qualified for a clinical diagnosis of insomnia—and for many of them, the problem began at age eleven.

And you know the most surprising finding of all? Most of their parents had no idea their kids had trouble getting enough sleep.[6]

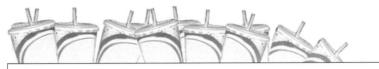

Fifty Ways to SuperSize Your Kids   #13

Let your children or teens sleep less than nine hours per night.

Despite the strong trend toward fewer sleeping hours, evidence is accumulating that *nine hours is the optimum amount of sleep for children and teens*. That means that if we want to give our kids the best chance of avoiding the physical devastation caused by carrying around too much weight, we need to make sure they get the rest they so desperately need. We need to teach them to make it a priority to R.E.S.T.—Reclaim Essential Sleep Time.

WHAT HAPPENS TO SLEEPLESS ADULTS?

While children are not adults, we have every reason to think that the same kinds of nasty things that plague adults who fail to get enough sleep will also afflict sleep-deprived children. And the news should alarm us.

While we were writing this chapter, news broke on a large-scale study of adults that found "a surprisingly strong link between the amount of shut-eye people get and their risk of becoming obese."[7] The study, presented at a meeting of the North American Association for the Study of Obesity, analyzed information from about eighteen thousand American adults who participated in the federal government's national Health and Nutrition Examination Survey throughout the 1980s. It revealed that adults who got less than four hours of sleep a night were 73 percent more likely to be obese than those who slept from seven to nine hours. Adults who averaged five hours of sleep had a 50 percent higher risk of obesity, while those who got six hours of sleep had a 23 percent higher chance.

In other words, the less sleep they got, the fatter they tended to be.

Why this strong link? Again, scientists aren't ready to pronounce a single definitive reason, but they have their suspicions. In general, sleep deprivation appears to damage the body's ability to determine how much food it needs. In more technical terms it lowers leptin, a blood protein that decreases appetite, so the less you sleep, the greater your appetite. Not getting enough sleep also raises levels of grehlin, a chemical that increases the urge to eat. So failure to sleep enough increases your yearning to eat food you don't need. A sleep deficit can also reduce the body's ability to process insulin and can interfere with your body's ability to regulate blood sugar, which can lead to a wide variety of health problems. The result? Sleepy people are prone to eat too much, quickly put on weight, and be at greater risk for poor health.

Dr. Rafael Pelayo of Stanford University's Sleep Disorder Clinic says reduced sleep can endanger your health in many other ways as well:

- Your ability to concentrate and remember fades.
- You can't think of the word you want.
- You get irritable.
- You become more prone to infections.
- You can even put yourself at risk for death.[8]

German researchers at the University of Lübeck concluded that well-rested people get a boost to their immune system that helps them better fight off attacking viruses than the sleep-deprived. They published their findings in the journal *Psychosomatic Medicine* and told the news organization Reuters, "Our results are amazing in that they show a decrease in antibody titer after only a single night of sleep deprivation."[9] In other words, the number of the body's infection-fighting "soldiers," the antibodies, significantly dropped with only one night of poor sleep.

Adults who don't get enough sleep suffer a marked slowing of reaction time. They have trouble paying sustained attention. They can't focus on multiple sources of information. They have higher cortisol levels, which tends to make them gain weight differently or gain more weight than individuals who get a proper amount of sleep. Their creativity plummets. Their brain seems to function in slow motion. They tend to experience "microsleeps," repeated intervals of one to ten seconds in which their brain processes no information at all.

Does the same type of thing happen to kids who don't get enough sleep? We have no reason to think it doesn't. When a child doesn't get enough sleep at night, he or she is likely to suffer from many consequences:

- More food is consumed during the day to try to stay alert.
- Hormones controlling appetite and weight won't work correctly.
- Some researchers believe that sleepy kids tend to resist insulin, which interferes with their ability to digest and process carbohydrates—which leads to weight gain.

And consider this: A 2004 Chinese study said that children who sleep less than seven hours a night increase their risk for suicide *threefold*.[10]

THE MAJOR ISSUE

Forget all the studies for a moment—or any of the mistakes you may have made in this area of sleep. Think about the problem in a simpler way.

Kids who have the opportunity to sleep late tend to do so. Kids who sleep late often don't have time for breakfast or don't feel like eating it. And kids who don't eat breakfast suffer a domino effect that can lead to weight gain and a decline in health.

Since they're starving by midmorning, they visit the vending machines, where they buy highly processed snacks. Their insulin levels soar as a result, and by the time they get to lunch, they're still hungry. Then they eat foods with a lot of sugar and fat, which results in sleepiness (negatively affecting school performance). This daytime sleepiness adds to the sleepiness they might already have from not enough sleep at night.

Sleepy kids find that their "get-up-and-go" has "got up and gone"! They don't have the energy or motivation to get involved in physical activity, so they put on weight, and the increased weight decreases their ability and desire to move. Tired and heavy children tend to feel much less motivated to exercise or play, and they usually have less endurance or physical stamina, so even if they did go out to play, chances are they would not exercise as long or as hard as they would have had they felt well rested.

And the more overweight the child is, the less he or she wants to move, in part because it hurts to move—overweight children suffer more back and joint pain than kids of healthy weight. That, in turn, disturbs their sleep and makes them even more tired.

And so the awful cycle goes on and on.

It's time we put a stop to it.

WHAT TO DO

Whatever methods you use to get your kids the sleep they need, keep one goal in mind: They usually require at least nine hours of sleep a night. Whatever you have to do to reach this goal, do it. You're the parent. You're the family's health care quarterback. Find some plays that work and use them. You might find the following suggestions helpful.

Cut Out the Caffeine

Did you know that caffeine can have a functional half-life of *six hours* in kids? In other words, half of the caffeine a child ingests at 3 P.M. will still be circulating in the body at 9 P.M., and a quarter of the caffeine will still remain in their system by 3 the next morning! Caffeine keeps them awake, so if you want your kids in bed by nine, you've got to cut off the chocolate, soda, cocoa, and anything else with caffeine in it by 3 or 4 P.M.

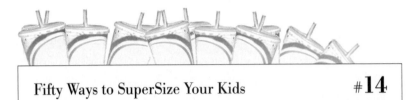

Fifty Ways to SuperSize Your Kids   #**14**

Let your kids have caffeinated drinks, cocoa, or chocolate after 3 P.M.

Pull the Plug

A study from the medical center at the University of Southwestern Texas recommended that TVs and computer monitors be turned off at least thirty minutes before a child goes to bed. It said the type of light emitted by a TV screen or computer monitor stimulates the child's brain and prevents the child from getting ready for sleep.

In addition, playing video games or watching television shows that feature chase scenes activates the system in the brain that creates wakefulness; kids who engage in those activities right before bed are going to have a tougher time falling asleep. So carefully watch the activities that occur one hour before your kids' bedtime. Give your children time before bed to think, relax, and get ready for sleep.

Set and Enforce Bedtime and Wake-up Hours

We think it's crucial for children to have regular bedtime and wake-up hours. When Walt's kids were little, his wife would begin the process by giving out reminders half an hour to forty-five minutes before bedtime. "It's 9:15," she might say, "so it's lights-out in forty-five minutes." And then fifteen minutes later, "It's 9:30, lights-out in thirty minutes." They didn't want to be telling their teens at 9:59, "Hey, you have to be in bed in one minute!"

They also talked and prayed together before the kids' bedtime. Walt considers this to be one of his family's most important bedtime routines. From their youngest years, either Barb or Walt would be at their children's bedside, spending that last five or ten or fifteen minutes to chat about whatever was on their minds. And then they prayed together before bed. So from their earliest years, bedtime prayer preceded lights-out. It became kind of a conditioned response.

Their daughter, Kate, is now twenty-six. Even today, when she visits and they have a little time of talk and prayer close to her bedtime, it's not unusual to see her yawn!

Did they allow exceptions to this practice? Of course. But in general, they thought the routine very important.

What can you do if you've never had such a practice? What if your child isn't used to a bedtime or wake-up routine? Begin by employing little steps. Consider wake-up time, for example. You might start by getting the child up at 7:30 A.M.; the next month you get him up a half hour earlier, at 7 A.M.; and the next month your target is 6:30 A.M. Set explicit, reasonable expectations and then enforce them. Make the changes in increments.

And understand that this is important not only for your children but also for you. In our experience the child who has been getting up at 8:05 A.M. to catch the 8:10 bus has a parent who has been getting up at 7:45 A.M. him- or herself. It really is a family issue. Ask yourself, "What are we doing as a family? How can we begin to change in such a way that it begins to improve our overall health?"

Getting up late is a learned habit. To change it, start taking some small steps to learn other, healthier habits. Things *can* change.

Food for Thought

Staying up late is a learned habit.

Teach your children disciplines that they can apply as they grow. As your kids mature, your role starts moving from parent to coach. Getting up earlier will allow you to have family time—and breakfast together as a family usually means going to bed early. Anything you can do to help your family get healthy will have benefits for years to come.

Establish a Regular Family Schedule

Beyond bedtime and wake-up time, a regular family schedule does wonders for a family's health. Children gain comfort and security from established routines and traditions. A consistent schedule tends to improve feelings of security and comfort even while it reduces anxiety and depression. A family schedule also helps kids to eat better; they know the times to expect breakfast, lunch, dinner and snacks.

When Walt's kids were little, they got used to a basic schedule. Whenever possible, they ate dinner together as a family and cleaned up as a family. If they had some TV time in the evening, they watched specific shows; they didn't use the remote control to flip through the options. And after watching, they tended to talk about what they saw.

Sherri grew up on a farm, where breakfast became the normal family meal together; her dad never knew when he would be coming in that evening. During breakfast they had worship and prayer times together and found out what was going on with everyone. She still considers it a wonderful tradition.

Maybe in your family, lunch is the family meal together. The key is to have as many meals together as possible.

Try not to become dictatorial or militaristic about the schedule you set, but do set one. Of course, you can vary your routine or decide as a family to deviate from it; but in general, it's beneficial for the entire family to have routines. Then evaluate those routines to see if they're helping to promote healthier lives.

"WE DID IT!"

As you read this chapter, did you find any surprises or things you could change? We hope you feel encouraged and equipped to help your children get the full night's sleep that they need to avoid becoming SuperSized (or to reduce their SuperSize status).

Once Walt learned about the importance of rest and what could be done to ensure a good night's sleep, he began to address this issue with his patients. One success story came from Betsy. In junior high Betsy participated in both cheerleading and gymnastics and had a very good BMI of 21. But over the next two years her BMI soared and her school performance sank. As her weight ballooned, her acne flared up. She dropped out of gymnastics and cheerleading, and the explosive combination of a widening figure and a blemished face led to teasing, bullying, and eventually depression.

Walt saw her just before her freshman year in high school. Other than her acne and weight, her physical exam and lab work came back normal. A depression screening test, however, did not. It came back positive.

When Walt talked with her, he learned she had some sloppy dietary habits. She engaged in no meaningful physical activity at all. And her parents had made the same mistake Walt had—they allowed her to have a TV in her bedroom. (More than half of parents report that their children have televisions in their bedrooms.[11] And 42 percent of children aged nine to seventeen have their own cable or satellite television hookups in their bedrooms.[12]) Not only that, but she had unfettered broadband Internet access in her bedroom and spent most of the late night watching TV and IM'ing "friends" all over the world.

By the time of her office visit, Betsy was averaging four hours of sleep a night—and she felt miserable. Fortunately she and her mom willingly decided to go to work together.

The first step: get the TV and Internet out of her bedroom. They agreed to set a specific bedtime and to get Betsy nine hours of sleep every night, not just on school nights. Both agreed to start a Weight Watchers program and to work out together at a local health club for the rest of the summer.

Betsy wanted to try out for the cheerleading squad the next spring. Walt agreed to hold them both accountable and to help Betsy clear up her acne ASAP.

Together, they made slow but sure progress. Despite some normal setbacks along the way, by the next spring, Betsy's BMI had shrunk from 26 to 23; her mom's had dropped from 29 to 26. Both felt in good physical and mental shape and had rewarded themselves with some new wardrobe items at Christmas.

Walt felt delighted for them both.

One afternoon while he was seeing patients, Tish, Walt's nurse, walked up to him. "There's someone who wants to see you, Dr. Larimore," she said. "I think it's important. Can you take a minute?"

"Sure," he replied, knowing that Tish would not interrupt patient flow unless she considered it significant. So Walt followed her up to the nurses' station. There sat Betsy and her mom. Before he could greet them, Betsy shot out of her chair like a rocket and nearly leaped into his arms.

"We did it!" she shouted. "We did it, Dr. Larimore!"

He felt a bit befuddled as she sobbed in his arms. Her mom's cheeks, streaked with happy tears, contrasted with Tish's beaming face.

"What'd we do?" he asked.

"We made the cheerleading squad!" she squealed.

Walt gave her a big hug. Then she stepped back a bit.

"Betsy," he began, "I'm so happy for you. Congratulations! But *we* didn't do this. You and your mom did! And you deserve to be very pleased with your efforts."

"But," Betsy objected, "we could not have done it without your advice. I never would have given up TV and the computer. I never would have started getting the rest I needed. I never would have begun eating right or exercising again."

Walt smiled. "Well, okay!" he conceded. "Maybe we did do it together. But you and your mom get the most credit, okay?"

With tears in her eyes, she nodded happily.

Walt still hears from Betsy and her mom. They've kept up the good habits they began more than ten years ago. They're both strong and healthy. Although it was a nice accomplishment to make the cheerleading squad, the *great* accomplishment is that Betsy and her mom worked together to un-SuperSize a teen headed toward disaster. Nutrition and exercise were important. Accountability was critical.

But R.E.S.T. was indispensable.

And it is for your kids, too.

SIMPLE STEPS THAT WORK

Children need nine hours of sleep per night. If your child is getting less than this, consider a few tips to get you started moving in the right direction:

- Begin with lights-out fifteen minutes earlier than usual (you'll probably encounter some resistance, but hang in there). Increase this gradually until your child gets the needed amount of sleep.
- It takes about half an hour for our brains and bodies to calm down and get ready for sleep. Turn off the TV, computer, or video game at least half an hour before bedtime. Take this opportunity to spend quiet time with your child.
- Don't forget that you, too, need to get to bed at the right time, so set an example for your children.
- Our schedules usually change drastically on the weekends, but keep in mind that we do much better when we go to bed at nearly the same time each evening. You may extend bedtime by a short amount, but don't give in to the temptation to let your children stay up hours later than usual.
- Remember that caffeine ingested four to six hours before bedtime might keep your kids up; physical exercise or activity within an hour of bedtime might do the same.

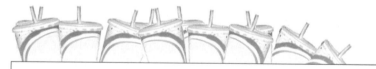

Fifty Ways to SuperSize Your Kids   #15

Let your kids go to bed as late as they want to. And let them watch TV right up until they go to bed.

7

FROM BOOB TUBE TO MEAN SCREEN

Walt met four-year-old Norm and his dad at a local church, where the boy's father served as pastor. Not too long afterward, Norm's mom began bringing him to Walt for his health care.

During one of his last well-child exams, Walt asked Norm, "What do you want to do when you grow up?"

He smiled and without a moment's hesitation exclaimed, "I want to be just like my dad!"

A few weeks after a final office visit, Norm's family moved out of town when his father got transferred to a church in another part of the state. Walt didn't see them again for five years. When they got reacquainted, Norm was nine years old and his family had just moved back to town . . . and Walt could hardly believe the change in his body.

Both Norm and his dad had ballooned into obese males. Indeed, Norm had become more like his dad than anyone could have imagined five years earlier.

Fortunately both the boy and his father felt ready to make some changes to improve their health. And Norm's mom, a fit and vivacious woman, was eager to help her struggling family.

Walt spent some time with each member of the family, going through an assessment very similar to the one discussed in Appendix A. To his surprise the biggest problems in each of their cases related to the amount of time they spent on the Internet, watching television, and playing video and Internet games.

When Norm's mom saw the evaluation, she nodded her head know-ingly. According to her, "Those boys are nearly addicted to video games! They play hours and hours and hours. And when it's not video games, they're watching sports events on TV. Often, when I'm going to bed, they are still going and going. They're like the Energizer Bunny when it comes to those games." She then lowered her head and contin-ued, "Dr. Larimore, I love the amount of time they spend together. I mean, they're best friends. But I'm concerned. Should I be?"

Maybe you're wondering the same thing. When it comes to the mean screen, how much is too much? And what about all those video games and all that time spent talking to friends on the computer? Could any of this be SuperSizing our kids?

Chances are, when your son or daughter mentions *Halo 2* or *Grand Theft Auto,* you have only a vague idea of what they're talking about. The fact is, the way we spend our leisure time has changed dra-matically in the past few decades. Most kids no longer go outside to play ball or ride bikes or hike to the local swimming hole. Nowadays they're much more likely to watch several hours of television, spend countless hours in front of the computer screen, play video game after video game, or lie on their beds and listen through headphones to a favorite hip-hop artist.

And the pounds just keep on coming.

A myriad relatively new entertainment options have made a sedentary lifestyle all too common among our youth. And most of this couch potato behavior starts right in front of the television set or computer screen.

RACKING UP THE HOURS

Most parents vastly underestimate the amount of television that their children watch, especially if those kids have a TV set in the bedroom.

A 2000 survey showed that the average American child spends about twenty-five hours a week in front of the television. Preschoolers watch twenty-eight hours of TV a week. That means a typical child watches 25,000 hours of television before his or her eighteenth birthday. Other surveys have found that nearly one out of every four children aged eight and older spend more than five hours a day watching TV and that children six and under spend an average of two hours a day watching television or playing computer and video games.

Food for Thought

The average American child spends nineteen to twenty-five hours a week in front of the TV.

According to the U.S. government, on average, children aged two to seventeen spend approximately 4.5 hours a day watching some kind of screen, with 2.5 to 2.75 hours of that amount spent on watching television. That's seventeen to nineteen hours a week in front of the TV! The table below shows the number of hours per day, on average, an American child spends glued to the boob tube.[1]

No matter who's taking the surveys, though, it quickly becomes clear that our kids are watching a lot of TV. And what's all that television watching doing to them, especially regarding their weight? The news could hardly be any worse.

THE NEGATIVE EFFECTS OF TV WATCHING

In Walt's experience most parents have no clue about how drastically television can harm their children's health. And that includes *all* aspects of their health.

As a parent himself, Walt wishes he had known that when his children sat in front of the television, physiological changes slowed down their metabolism and increased their appetite. Children who eat in front of the TV—any kind of eating, snacks or meals—especially in a reclined position, eat much more than they would if they sat at the

Total Screen Media per Day

TV, Video Games, Computers, Videos/DVDs Combined

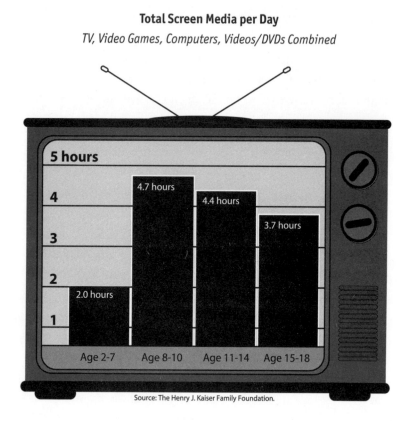

Source: The Henry J. Kaiser Family Foundation.

dinner table. In addition, the types of foods they eat in front of the television tend to be more processed, higher in saturated fat and sugars, and nutritionally barren.

Researchers have found fairly direct correlations between the amount of time a child spends in front of the TV and the risk and degree of obesity he or she faces. One study showed that children who watch five or more hours of television per day are five times more likely to be overweight or obese than those who watch less than two hours per day.

The data are so compelling that the American Academy of Pediatrics recommends that children over the age of two watch no more than two hours of *any* kind of television, even educational programs.

Recipe for Success

The American Academy of Pediatrics recommends that children over the age of two watch no more than two hours per day of *any* kind of television.

And for children under two, it recommends no television exposure at all.

But let's get more specific. What kind of harm can excessive TV viewing cause your kids? Get ready for a shock.

Food for Thought

According to Harvard University's long-running Nurses' Health Study of fifty thousand women, for every two hours of TV a person watches, the risk of becoming obese jumps 23 percent, while the risk of developing diabetes increases 14 percent.[2]

General Effects

- The Framingham Children's Study found that preschool children who watched the most TV had the greatest increases in body fat by adolescence. The negative impact of watching TV was even greater for preschool children who were sedentary or had a diet higher in fat.[3]
- Children and adolescents who watch too much TV may experience early-onset puberty. Scientists from Mayer Hospital at the University of Florence discovered that children who didn't watch television for a full week and instead played sports, read books, and got active in other ways experienced a 30 percent jump in their levels of melatonin, the hormone thought to prevent early puberty. Lead study author Robert Salti theorized that the light and radiation emitted from TV and computer screens

disturb the production of melatonin, which regulates the body's internal clock.[4]

- The amount of television a child watches corresponds directly to the risk of developing serious health problems as an adult. Television viewing between the ages of five and fifteen years increases the risk of high cholesterol levels, smoking, poor fitness, and being overweight in adulthood. "Our results suggest that excessive television viewing in young people is likely to have far-reaching consequences for adult health," the authors of a study concluded. "We concur with the American Academy of Pediatrics that parents should limit children's viewing to one to two hours per day; in fact, data suggest that less than one hour a day would be even better."[5]

- A study of more than one thousand children between the ages of two and twelve revealed that children who watch two to four hours of TV a day have a significantly higher likelihood of high cholesterol levels and obesity than those who watch less than two hours a day.[6]

- Children who watch TV tend to burn fewer calories per minute than children involved in almost any other activity—not only fewer than those engaged in active play but also fewer than those who read or "do nothing." In fact, the child watching TV burns almost as few calories as a sleeping child—and the heavier the child, the more grave the effect. For children of normal weight, TV watching triggers a 12 percent drop in metabolism. Obese children have a 16 percent drop in metabolism. Lead researcher Dr. Robert Klesges concluded, "It seems prudent for people of all ages who have weight problems to curb their time in front of the tube and do something more demanding instead."[7]

- The more television children watch, the fewer fruits and vegetables they eat, perhaps because the advertising they see leaves them craving junk food instead.[8]

- Children who watch too much TV have lower creativity, increased weight and blood pressure, decreased family interaction, lower school performance, and more sociopathic behavior.

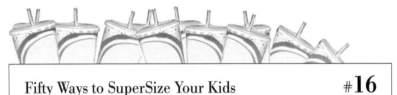

Fifty Ways to SuperSize Your Kids   #16

Allow your kids to watch all the TV they want.

A Passive Occupation

The basic problem is that TV is a passive occupation, a sedentary pastime. Kids watching TV aren't just sedentary physically; they're sedentary mentally and relationally. Kids who watch too much television not only burn few calories, they even burn fewer calories than if they were sitting at the kitchen table doing homework. Plus, the more TV a child watches, the less he or she exercises. And that compounds the problem.

With passivity also comes shorter attention spans, and TV reflects this shift. If you were to go back and watch *The Jetsons* or *Bonanza* or *I Love Lucy*, you would see scenes that last up to ninety seconds or more. Dad comes home; the shot stays on him and the cameraman pulls back to show the whole living room. The entire scene might last up to two minutes without a single camera cutaway. But watch TV shows today and you won't see a shot that lasts more than eight seconds.

When CNN Headline News started broadcasting on January 1, 1982, viewers saw only a single news anchor sitting at a desk. Now you see one or two anchors, headlines behind the anchor, and one or two headlines streaming across the screen below the anchor.

TV scenes and Internet pop-ups change so quickly because of shorter attention spans. And if your attention span is shrinking, it makes it just that much easier to sit there and eat a whole bag of chips without realizing what you're doing.

Dr. Jane M. Healy, an educational psychologist, coined a phrase we like: "the Two-Minute Mind." She means that our brains are becoming impatient with anything that requires depth of processing. The mentally passive medium of TV tends to create this mind. Watching TV develops brain circuits with much shorter attention spans.

Eating in Front of the TV

The American Dietetic Association has discovered that not only do parents underestimate the amount of time a child spends watching television, they also imagine that their kids are not eating in front of the TV. But when the children are asked, they reply, "We almost always eat when we watch TV." It's a triple whammy: The kids are not moving because they're planted in front of the TV, they're not exercising as much for the same reason, and, to top it off, they're snacking more.

A study of third and fifth graders at California public schools found that, on average, elementary school children consumed roughly 20 percent of their daily calories while watching TV. And on the weekends kids munched more than one-quarter of their calories for the day while watching TV. They also tended to eat fewer fruits and vegetables and more soda and fast food while the TV roared on.[9]

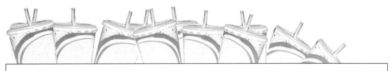

Fifty Ways to SuperSize Your Kids   #17

Permit your kids to eat or snack in front of the TV or keep the TV on during mealtime.

In addition, when families eat in front of the television, they lose all the benefit of family interaction. Study after study has shown that the more meals a family shares together—with the TV off—the better health those children enjoy. No matter how bad nutritionally the meals are, in general they tend to be better than if the family eats out or if it eats in front of the TV. The more TV a family watches, the more likely its members are to ingest foods high in bad fat and salt. And the more TV a family watches, the more likely everyone is to drink sugar-laden drinks like soda pop.

Ads Aimed at Kids

Did you know that the typical child sees about forty thousand commercials a year on TV, most of them for candy, cereal, soda, and fast food? The food and beverage industries spend $10 billion or more a year marketing directly to children and youth.[10]

Food for Thought

Most of the TV ads directed at children promote high-calorie foods and beverages, such as candy, snack foods, fast foods, soft drinks, and sweetened breakfast cereals.

Advertising executives design commercials to impact kids and even skew the way kids influence their parents' buying decisions. Ads targeted at children virtually always showcase the most unhealthy foods and food types available, whether for sugar-laden cereals or fatty fast foods. A 2000 study showed that 80 percent of all advertisements aired during children's programs pitch unhealthful foods![11]

Not all of these commercials targeting our kids come via the boob tube. Many advertisers are starting to use the Internet to market their foods to children. At KidzTown.com, Hershey's offers a "Twizzlers Slider" puzzle. Nabiscoworld.com has a mini golf challenge in which children try to sink a ball while avoiding a Ritz Bits sandwich. This site attracts 800,000 children monthly; kids spend an average of twelve minutes per visit.

Elizabeth Vandewater, an expert on human development at the University of Texas in Austin, said this about commercial messages geared toward kids: "We know that advertising works, and it works well." Psychologist Dale Kunkel of the University of California at Santa Barbara agrees. "It works especially well on young children," he said.[12] Do you think it's any coincidence that the high-sugar cereals advertised on Saturday mornings get shelved in the supermarket at the eye level of a three-year-old? Advertisers know that if they can get Junior to tug on Mommy's leg, those Triple Sugar Donutios will make their way into the shopping cart. Their advertising *works*.

Did you know that in 2002, advertisers spent about $12 *billion* targeting our children? Children who watched Saturday morning TV viewed more than twice as many ads for unhealthful foods as adults did on programs aired after 9 P.M. A 2001 study found nearly 95 percent of all the foods advertised during kids' programs were for fast food, sugary cereals, soft drinks, and candy.[13] And the numbers only rise each year.

With figures like these in mind, Sweden and Norway have banned junk-food advertising to children, and Great Britain is considering the same move. Why don't we? Good question, and we'll talk more about that in Chapter 13, "Battle of the Bulge on the Statehouse Steps."

Don't be fooled! If your kids watch a lot of TV or spend a lot of time on the Internet, it's working on *them*, too.

RACKING UP STILL MORE HOURS— AND PAYING FOR IT

How much time do our kids spend online or playing video games? We have less data for that than we do for television viewing, but without question the amount of time is increasing. And too many hours spent on these activities does our children no more good than watching too much TV.

Food for Thought

For every hour a child plays video games, he or she can double his or her risk of obesity.

Did you know that for every hour a child plays video games or watches television, he or she may double his or her risk of obesity? Nicolas Stettler, pediatric nutrition specialist at the Children's Hospital of Philadelphia, concluded in one study, "Our findings suggest that the use of electronic games should be limited to prevent childhood obesity."[14] And did you know that children with a higher BMI spend more time playing video games than children in the same age group with lower BMIs?[15]

Consider, too, that these games can become addicting, particularly for certain children. The makers of these games do a couple of very interesting things to keep the kids coming back for more. For one, they're making them increasingly lewd and violent, at deeper and deeper levels—levels most parents will never reach. If a parent were to sit down to play the game on his or her own, he or she would probably reach only the second or third level, and so may see nothing terribly objectionable; but the designers have created the game so that a player does not get to the violent or depraved material until level six or seven or even further in. Second, the Internet versions of these games, in particular, never end. They literally go on and on, just as *Dungeons and Dragons* pulled kids into spending countless hours on its dark fantasies back in the late eighties and early nineties.

To be sure, some recent video games are trying to get kids up and moving. Dance Dance Revolution is one such example. Players place a touch-sensitive pad on the floor, and while music plays, footprints come up on the video screen, showing players which steps to make on the footpads. The game became quite popular at arcades and quickly went to a home version. Another game features virtual-reality boxing. Kids put on a pair of wired gloves, stand in front of a video screen, and throw punches; the game mimics the punches they throw. When a player ducks, his counterpart on the screen ducks; when a child moves to the side or jumps, his video persona does the same. After one game of three or four rounds, kids often come away drenched in sweat.

Other games try to get kids to eat better (no, we're not kidding). Squire's Quest, for example, is a computer game developed by Baylor

College of Medicine's Children's Nutrition Research Center. It tries to teach kids to eat more fruits and vegetables. Kids can advance in the game by learning how to talk to their parents about serving orange juice at breakfast.

While these games represent a little improvement, Walt has always tried to encourage parents to involve their children in exercise or activity that's *relational,* person-to-person. That way, the activity not only tones a child's body and mind but also helps tone the child emotionally and relationally.

Are these new kinds of games better than nothing? Absolutely. But children who play *together* tend to develop better social skills. They learn to negotiate, to share, to communicate, and to prioritize—and they won't learn those kinds of skills by engaging in a solitary activity.

SO WHAT CAN WE DO?

While we could suggest dozens of ways to help cage the effects of the mean screen in your house and get your kids headed in a better direction, let's start with just five possible courses of action. Pick one, see how it goes, and then at a later time try some others. The key is to take at least *one* positive action today!

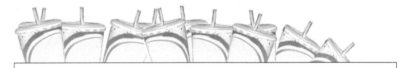

Fifty Ways to SuperSize Your Kids   #18

Give your child unrestricted TV and Internet access in his or her bedroom.

1. Take the TV and Computer out of Your Child's Room

Do you know one common result of taking the television out of a child's room? That child's weight tends to go down.

If your child has a television in his or her room, take it out. And if you have a TV in your own bedroom, be a good example and take it out as well. Kids learn more by example than they do by preaching. So practice what you preach, Mom and Dad.

"But the television helps my kids settle down after a long day," you may object. "I'll never get them in their rooms if they don't have the TV in there."

We hate to contradict you, but the University of Texas Southwestern Medical Center has found that watching TV and working on a computer—two activities that parents tend to believe calm down their children before bedtime—actually rouse children instead. The bright lights of the TV and computer screen actually stimulate the brain. So the center recommends turning off the TV and computer at least thirty minutes before your child's bedtime to give those young brains time to wind down.

And here's another little tidbit: Having a TV in a preschool child's bedroom increases the risk of obesity even more than TV viewing alone.

Because most children begin viewing TV before the age of two, parents need to be educated about the importance of removing the television, computer, and game console from every child's bedroom.[16]

2. Keep All Forms of Entertainment in a Central Location

Imagine that it's 10 o'clock on a cold, rainy night. You hear a knock at the door, so you get up, flip on the porch light, and see a grungy, dirty, unshaven, cigar-smoking guy with a raincoat and a tattered hat just outside your door. He looks kind of suspicious and shifty-eyed, so you only open the door a crack and say, "May I help you?"

"Yeah," he replies, "I'm here to see your kids. I was just wondering if I could go back in the bedroom and spend some time with them."

What parent in his or her right mind would consider doing anything other than slamming the door and calling the police? You wouldn't even *think* about letting that creepy stranger into your kids' bedrooms.

But when we allow our children to have a TV or unfettered Internet access or a game console in their bedrooms, that is exactly what we're doing. We're allowing people who do not have our children's best interests at heart to have direct access to our kids.

If you choose to have Internet and television and video games in your home, then at least keep them in a public location. That way, both parents and children have family accountability. Don't allow potentially dangerous electronic strangers to hang out in your child's bedroom!

3. Don't Eat in Front of the TV

If you choose to have a TV in your home, then by all means make sure that you don't eat in front of it. Make that a forbidden activity, except possibly for those rare occasions when it might make sense—a Super Bowl party, for example, or a gathering to watch a significant show. But in general, during food preparation time and eating meals, the TV and computer and all video games should remain off.

4. Have Appropriate Snacks Available

If you decide to have a movie night or Super Bowl party or something like it, then make sure you have some healthy snacks around the house (see Chapter 10, "Gearing Up for Healthy Family Meals," for suggestions). You want your teens to be able to come to your house, hang out, and enjoy themselves, not feel like they're in prison. Consider these events as opportunities to teach your children not only how to snack appropriately and in a healthy way but also the other kids who visit. Make it a fun time, a healthy time, and a memorable time—not a big drag.

5. Try a TV-Free Night (or Week)

The research of Barbara Brock at Eastern Washington University shows that television-free families—even if they keep the television off only once a week—have better relationships within the family.[17] They're more likely to have sit-down dinners and family activities together and to engage in hobbies, games, chores, pet care, walking, music, gardening, community service, housecleaning, outdoor activities, and writing—all of which burn more calories than watching TV.

Food for Thought

Parents in television-free homes have about an hour of meaningful conversation every day with their children, compared to a national average of five to seven minutes in other homes.[18]

Parents in television-free homes have about an hour of meaningful conversation every day with their children, compared to a national average of five to seven minutes in other homes.[19] Nearly 70 percent of parents feel their children got along better without their television; nearly 70 percent of parents have also reported they had not only more time with their children but more mealtimes together.

Children in television-free homes tend to be more active physically than other children of their age. One-quarter of the TV-free children studied kept physically active thirteen or more hours per week. Such increased activity obviously helps children tone up and keep weight off. Only 7 percent of television-free children are ten or more pounds overweight, and less than two in one hundred have an eating disorder.

To us, that's stunning information.

It's also interesting that the computer and Internet do not take over TV's role in most TV-free homes. Although 98 percent of television-free homes own a computer, many television-free children actually report more boredom with computer and video games than their television-crippled friends.[20]

Contrary to what one might think, children in television-free homes aren't missing out on anything. Brock writes, "The vast majority of responses indicate that TV-watching families are the ones missing out on life."

If you decide to have one TV-free night per week (or one week per month), you need to come up with a plan about what you're going to do instead. If you decide that on Tuesday nights you're not watching TV, but you have no plan for what you're going to do, your kids are not going to sit there and twiddle their thumbs. So brainstorm about what your family might like to do. What games do you like to play? What books could you read together? What nearby park could you visit? It's important that your kids have something available ahead of time that they really like to do. Otherwise, it's just too easy to turn on the TV.

What do families who have TV-free time do? They interact with each other. They find other activities that they enjoy doing as a family. Even card games or board games stimulate much more brain activity than just vegging out in front of the TV.

Focus on the Family has a series of resources about family nights and how to make them fun and help kids remember lessons for life (see www.SuperSizedKids.com for details). Parents can take the time that they would have spent in front of the TV—literally time thrown away—and instead have fun with their kids.

Maybe it becomes a family date night. It might be nothing more than going to the library; but it ought to be something that puts you together with your kids in a fun and productive atmosphere. Whatever you choose, replace highly sedentary behavior (which results in obesity and poor eating habits) with activity that's more likely to generate a higher quality of family life and better eating habits.

The TV-free movement sponsors a national TV-free week and runs a nice Web site. (You can learn more about this at our own Web

site, www.SuperSizedKids.com.) It offers loads of easy, doable suggestions that can get a family on its way. Start small and work your way
up! You might be surprised what time without a television might do
for your family.

Shortly after a series of powerful hurricanes raked Florida in 2004,
Sherri was listening to a call-in program on a local radio station.
People phoned in to report positive experiences brought about by the
storms. One girl identified herself as twelve years old and said that
because her house's electricity remained off for three or four days,
her family actually spent some significant time together. They sat
down and played games, they talked to each other. Without electricity
they couldn't watch TV. And she loved it.

Dr. Tom Robinson, a pediatrician at Stanford University, studies
obesity. He wanted to see if reducing the amount of TV that kids
watched helped them to drop pounds. It did. Two of his studies, on a
total of eleven hundred children aged eight to ten, showed that by
reducing television watching, even the children who got heavier
gained less weight. Robinson discovered that turning off the television
slowed down obesity more than anything else, including exercise programs and diets. "It amazed me that we saw these effects," he said.[21]

Why don't you let it amaze you, too, in your own home?

YOU CAN STOP THE LOSING STREAK

Our kids are gaining weight like never before, and much of that
weight gain comes down to a simple equation:

more TV + more junk food – exercise = SuperSized Kids

Soon it becomes a vicious cycle. Their weight balloons while their
physical, mental, and relational health declines.

Do you remember the story that began this chapter—the story of
Norman, the preacher's kid? It has a very good ending.

Norman and his parents, along with his older brother and sister, decided to give the boob tube the boot. After reading about TV-free homes they decided to join the movement.

Not only did the TV go, but so did the video games. Norman reported, "I had more fun going out and throwing a football or kicking a soccer ball with my dad than we ever did watching overpaid athletes do the same. Dad and I began shooting hoops together. We walked and even began jogging together. We had fun getting fit, and our relationship is stronger than ever!"

The family also moved all their computers into one room and use them only for e-mail and research. "No more IMs for me!" declared Norman.

Slowly at first, almost imperceptibly, the weight began to fall off both Norman and his dad. And now, nearly a decade later, they are still big men—but their BMIs are much closer to normal than ever before.

But there's even more. Norm's dad summed it up this way: "Our family's health was going down for the count. I'm glad we were able to break the vicious cycle that I allowed to start in my family!"

As your children's health care quarterback, it's up to you to stop the losing streak. You have to take control of the entertainment options under your roof and make sure that they quit harming your kids. Super-Sized time in front of the mean screen, more times than not, results in SuperSized Kids—and that's not a winning record for anybody.

SIMPLE STEPS THAT WORK

Encourage, enable, and expect your children to spend less time in front of the TV. At first blush this may seem like an impossible task. But it will reap huge health benefits. The goal is two hours or less of TV, computer, and video games (combined) daily. This doesn't have to be accomplished overnight; instead, take small steps to get from where your child is to where you want him or her to be. Consider these tips:

- Sit down as a family and decide which shows you will watch during the coming week. Let each child have a say so that everyone feels part of this decision and will more likely go along with the new plan.

■ Get TVs and unfettered Internet out of the bedrooms. Discuss why they should be taken out and set a date for their removal. This will give everyone time to adjust. Parents, if you have a TV in your room, set an example and remove yours, too.

■ Try to make passive TV watching more active. Have a contest to see who can jump rope or keep a hula hoop going the longest during commercials. Use your imagination and come up with fun contests that involve movement.

■ Learn more about TV-free weeks. Consider trying a TV-free week each year, then every three months, then a week a month. Before you know it, your family may be completely TV-free. (You can find more information on TV-free homes at www. SuperSizedKids.com.)

■ If computer time unrelated to schoolwork is an issue in your home, set a kitchen timer on top of the monitor and tell your child that his/her time is up when the bell rings.

■ Set up a system where your child can "buy" fifteen minutes of extra computer time by walking the dog, riding his bike an extra fifteen minutes, mowing the lawn (only if you have a push mower), or playing basketball.

■ If you allow video games in your home, try to find those that teach good habits. And be sure you find a reputable review of any game your child considers buying. We have tips for you at www.SuperSizedKids.com.

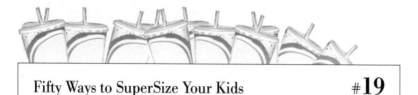

Fifty Ways to SuperSize Your Kids   #**19**

Allow your kids to play video games as much as they want to.

8

GET UP, GET OUT, GET FUN, GET FIT

A few years ago some family friends of Sherri's moved to the Orlando area. Their sixth-grade son, Bobby, seemed to support the move and appeared to enjoy the change in his surroundings . . . all except for one thing. At his new school he quickly ran headlong into a big challenge—quite literally.

The school required all sixth graders to go outside every day and run around the school yard. Because Bobby was the typical sixth grader and weighed a few more pounds than he should, he hated that run. He wasn't good at it. It winded him easily.

And he always came in dead last.

IT MIGHT BE HARD TO GET STARTED

If you have a child like Bobby who struggles with weight and related health issues and you want to help him or her to get up and get moving to drop some of those unwanted pounds, first we want to say, "Great! It's one of the best possible ways you can help your child."

But immediately after that, we'd like to give you a caution.

Remember this: A SuperSized child has a lot of trouble just getting started. It's very hard for kids like these to get going, to get active, and to get some exercise. They face extraordinary challenges on at least three levels.

Physical challenges. Their excess weight makes them less flexible and more likely to suffer aches and pains; and the more they move, the more aches and pains they feel. They have up to five times more fat cells and less functional muscle. And so they struggle to perform tasks their normal-weight peers find relatively easy.[1] Obese teens and even preteens may already suffer with arthritis or serious back problems that make it really hard, even painful, for them to get up and get started.

Emotional challenges. SuperSized Kids are more likely than others to be bullied, mocked, kidded, and insulted by total strangers, let alone by people they know. They will get stared at. That's extremely tough for young kids, because image is so important to them. So they tend to think, *Why should I go outside and exercise and invite the kind of abuse I've already received?*

Relational challenges. Study after study has shown that obese kids have much more difficulty making and sustaining healthy relationships than kids of normal weight. We wish we could say that the fat, friendless kid is a myth, but he's not. And the lonelier these kids feel, the more likely they are to retreat from the relationships they already have and instead try to find solace in food—probably in front of the TV. Besides that, relationships within the family may make it harder for an obese child to lose weight and get healthy. Grandma may see those extra pounds as a sign of good health and may therefore offer donuts or sweets to the child without the parent's knowledge.

Yes, it's critical that we get our SuperSized Kids up and moving, but we have to realize that it won't be easy and it won't be quick.

Walt will never forget Stuart and his family. When it became clear that Stuart absolutely had to shed dozens of pounds, he and his family began walking together. One day shortly after they started this new, health-promoting habit, someone in a passing car shouted out an insult about Stuart's size. Stuart stopped dead in his tracks, his shoulders stooped, and all the wind rushed out of his sails.

But Stuart had something going for him: a wonderful mom. Instantly she recognized how the nasty remark had cut deep into her son's soul. She responded by physically turning Stuart to face her. Then she looked him eyeball-to-eyeball and said, "Stuart, what they don't see is the Stuart inside of you. That's what I see. Let's find him." And then the family continued its walk.

Weeks after this incident the family returned to Walt's office for a follow-up visit. Stuart had begun losing weight, he felt better physically, and his school performance had shot way up. "Do you think that's just a coincidence?" his mom asked.

"No," Walt replied, "I don't think it's a coincidence at all."

Food for Thought

When SuperSized Kids get active and improve their health-related habits, the positive results affect their physical, emotional, mental, and relational health.

When SuperSized kids get moving and on a more healthy track, the positive results ripple into every area of their lives. They feel better about themselves. They find new self-confidence. Their self-image improves. They sleep better. They become less withdrawn. They perform better in school (more on that in Chapter 11, "Be Part of the School Solution"). Regular exercise has been linked to a reduced risk of cancer, heart disease, diabetes, and high blood pressure.[2] And on and on the enormous benefits go.

Parents, we applaud you for wanting to get your kids to exercise more. Keep it up! But remember that if you have a SuperSized Kid, it's physically hard, emotionally hard, and relationally hard for him or her to get up and moving. You can't simply tell obese children to "go exercise." Not only is it really tough for them to do so, but they're likely to get knocked down once they try. You need to understand this hard fact and get ready for it.

If you have a SuperSized child, remember that he or she *has* to start slow. Don't make that first step impossible or even difficult to take! And if you have one child who's obese and another who's overweight, realize that it's going to be easier for the overweight child to get started than it will be for the obese child.

Don't let the difficulty of the task, however, stop you from taking that first step. Consider it carefully, plan for it wisely, encourage it positively—and then *get started*. Don't worry if it feels as if you're going too slowly. Just get started.

Recipe for Success

The only way things will ever get better is if you and your child get up and take that first step together.

GET OUT AND GET ACTIVE

You might be surprised to learn how motivated your children will become to "get out and get active" if they observe their parents— you—getting out and getting active. According to movement specialist Jane Clark, professor and chairwoman of the University of Maryland's Department of Kinesiology, "If a mother and father both exercise, compared to those who don't, kids in that house are six times more likely to exercise. If one parent exercises, the child is three times more likely."[3]

Do you want your child to get up and get active? If so, the best thing you can do by far is to get up and get active yourself.

And how much activity are we talking about? The recommendations vary slightly from group to group and from expert to expert, but most authorities recommend that both you and your child get at least sixty minutes a day of moderate to vigorous exercise—the kind of physical movement that can get your blood rushing, your lungs pumping, and your metabolism rising. Sixty minutes a day should be your *minimum* goal—and it doesn't have to be sixty minutes all at one time.

Specifically the National Association for Sport and Physical Education recommends at least 150 minutes of exercise per week for elementary school kids and 225 minutes per week for middle and high school kids.

The Centers for Disease Control and Prevention has adopted two recommendations. It says that elementary school children should accumulate at least thirty to sixty minutes of a variety of age-appropriate and developmentally appropriate physical activity on all or most days of the week. It says that some of the child's activity each day should come in periods lasting ten to fifteen minutes or more and include moderate to vigorous activity. It warns against children having extended periods of inactivity.

The CDC gives a separate recommendation for adolescents. It counsels that all adolescents should be physically active daily or nearly every day, as part of play, games, sports, work, transportation, recreation, physical education, or planned exercise. It particularly recommends that they get their exercise with family members, school friends, or as a part of community activities. Adolescents should engage in three or more sessions per week, it says, of vigorous to moderate activities that last twenty minutes or more at a time.

Sherri usually recommends that her clients exercise daily. She doesn't tell them, "At the end of the week you should have accumulated this much," since she knows human nature. Many of us would try to get all of that exercise in one or two days, without moving the rest of the week! "Well, I don't feel like doing it today," we tend to say, "but I still have five days left." But that won't work! Daily movement is best.

Recipe for Success

Help your kids find physical activity that is fun to do, that they enjoy doing, and then encourage them to find someone to do it with.

How can you and your child start to get up and get active if that hasn't been your practice? Allow us to offer a few suggestions.

Turn Off the TV

We've said it before, and we'll say it again: At the top of our list is turning off the TV and computer. Neither you nor your child will get up and get active if you don't first turn off the television set; so as your first active move, hit the off button. But remember, there's also a practical side to cutting back on your TV viewing. You need to have a good idea of what you're going to do instead of watching the tube. Don't turn off the TV in the living room and head to the computer or stereo in the bedroom! When you turn off the TV, have a clear plan in mind of what you and your child are going to do to get up and get active.

Don't Make Them Exercise Alone

It won't work to tell your child to go out alone and get some exercise. Children need to exercise with others whose company they enjoy. First on that list ought to be you: What kinds of physical activity could you do together that both you and your child would enjoy? Friends and other family members can also join in on the fun, the more the merrier. Health-promoting activities are easier to do in groups than alone, and the social aspect of the activity makes it more likely that you and your child will stick with it. Relationships build in such settings, and it's easier to get the exercise you need, since you don't get so focused on the exercise itself.

Consider a few other small suggestions for getting up and getting started:

- Work in the yard together.
- Walk or run to the mailbox together.
- Take a family walk before a meal together.

- Shoot some hoops, throw a ball, kick a soccer ball together.
- Plan weekend outings or vacations that involve physical activity.
- Go hiking or boating or rappelling together.

Families who get up and get active together often make a surprising discovery: The kids start enjoying it before the parents do, so the youngsters become great motivators for their elders to remain active.

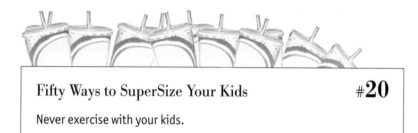

Fifty Ways to SuperSize Your Kids   #**20**

Never exercise with your kids.

The National Institutes of Health has its own recommendations for those who want to get up off the couch and start moving.[4] Consider how you can make their suggestions appropriate for your child:

Start very light. Increase your standing activities and special chores such as room painting, pushing a wheelchair, yard work, ironing, cooking, or playing a musical instrument.

Bump it up. Once you're comfortable moving your body, start with some slow walking, do some garage work, carpentry, housecleaning, child care, golf, sailing, or table tennis.

Bump it up some more. Get into moderate activity such as brisk walking, weeding and hoeing a garden, carrying a load, cycling, skiing, tennis, or dancing.

Keep moving. Eventually move into speed walking or walking with small weights uphill. Participate in sports such as basketball or soccer, flexibility exercises, strength or resistance training, and aerobic conditioning.

Self-monitor. Observe and record your calorie intake, servings of fruits and vegetables, exercise sessions, and medication usage. Set specific, attainable, and forgiving goals for yourself.

Pats on the Back

Give yourself rewards for meeting your goals. Treat yourself to a movie, buy a CD, put money away for a more costly item you want, take an afternoon off from work, or give yourself an hour of quiet time away from family.

And once more we would add: *Don't* treat yourself or your child with a big piece of cake or another fatty dessert!

Make Time to Exercise

Last, beware of the number one excuse for not getting up and getting active: "We're just too busy." When asked why we don't get up and get active for at least twenty minutes a day—active enough to produce an increase in heart or breathing rate—most of us reply, "I just don't have the time."

Listen, your health and the health of your children are at stake. If you don't feel as though you have the time to exercise, then take a good long look at your schedule and see what you can cut out in order to make time for getting up and getting active. And then make a promise to yourself that you'll never again say, "I'm just too busy." You aren't, and neither is your child.

GET FUN AND GET FIT

Throughout this chapter we've been using the word "exercise," but if you want to get your kids up and moving, it might be better to stay away from the e-word. Instead of saying, "Let's go get some exercise," try something more along the lines of, "Hey, would you like to go outside and shoot a few hoops?"

In other words, make it fun. And give them a choice. Encourage your kids to use their creativity in their choice of activities. Maybe they could make big paper airplanes and chase them around the yard, or perhaps on a trip to the beach they could build a fancy castle using sand and stones from a distance away.

And how about adding some music to the movement? Researchers from Ohio State University discovered that exercising to music may actually increase a person's brainpower. They found that cardiac rehabilitation patients who listened to music while working out increased their scores on a verbal fluency test. Charles Emery, a professor of psychology at OSU and the lead author of the study, said, "The combination of music and exercise may stimulate and increase the cognitive arousal while helping to organize cognitive output." Get rid of the professor-speak, and essentially he means that exercising to music might make both you and your kids smarter.[5]

Here's the main thing: *Make it fun and make it a habit.* Don't try to stick your kids with a regimented exercise program. They'll hate it, you'll hate it, and then you'll all be back to the TV.

Consider a few other simple suggestions for getting fun and getting fit.

Take a Walk

Did you know that people who take at least 10,000 steps a day are more likely than their more sedentary friends to have a healthy body weight, less body fat, and a smaller waist? That's the word from a study conducted at the University of Tennessee.[6] Since even sedentary children will often take 4,000 to 5,000 steps a day just walking around, and since a child can easily walk at a pace of about 100 steps per minute, if you and your child start walking for about thirty minutes a day (even if in three separate ten-minute periods), you'll get pretty close to that 10,000-step goal.

> Recipe for Success
>
> If you walk 2,000 steps a day more than you usually do, you'll never gain another pound.

Researchers at the Center for Human Nutrition at the University of Colorado Health Sciences Center claim that if you walk 2,000 steps a day more than you usually do, you'll never gain another pound. That even includes, for example, steps taken while pacing during a telephone conversation.[7]

A study reported in the *American Journal of Public Health* said that walking briskly for thirty minutes a day, or at a slower pace for sixty minutes a day, can more than burn off the hundred unneeded calories that many people take in daily. Another study, conducted at Duke University, found that participants who walked briskly for thirty minutes a day maintained their weight and some even lost a few pounds.[8] And researchers at Germany's University of Ulm Medical Center reported that walking just two hours a week could cut the risk of heart disease in half, compared with a sedentary person.

And what is a "brisk" walk? Edward Gregg, an epidemiologist with the CDC, says that "people should be able to carry on a conversation but know that their breathing is elevated." In other words, you and your child should be able to talk, but probably not be able to easily sing the national anthem.

And what does a brisk walk do for you other than keep your weight down or even help you to lose some pounds? It increases the efficiency of the heart. It improves lung capacity and breathing efficiency. It helps to lower blood pressure. It tends to lower the risk of stroke, heart disease, diabetes, and osteoporosis. It helps you sleep better and reduces your appetite. And it does wonders to improve mood. "If everyone in the U.S. were to walk briskly thirty minutes a day," said Dr. JoAnn Manson, chief of preventive medicine at Harvard's Brigham and Women's Hospital, "we could cut the incidence of many chronic diseases [by] thirty percent to forty percent."

So go for a walk and make a game out of it. Where in the world would you like to visit someday? Pick a destination, such as Paris or Rome, and figure out how many miles it is from where you live. Then translate that distance into a number of steps (use a pedometer to see how many steps you take over a mile course). Once you know the total number of steps it would take to walk there (forget for a moment that you'd have to walk on water), then you and your family can start walking your way to Paris or Rome, or Boise or Walla Walla—whatever destination you had in mind. Once you "reach" your destination, treat the walkers to a reward—maybe a favorite CD or a deposit into the family vacation fund. This is a novel way to get the whole family involved. And you don't have to think about Rome or Paris! Maybe the whole family wants to visit a place just sixty miles away. You can keep track of your steps using a basic pedometer, and many manufacturers make pedometers just for kids, in neon colors and unusual, fun shapes.

The CDC has developed a program called Kids Walk to School that shows parents how to organize a safe walk-to-school program. (We'll talk more about this in Chapter 11, and you can find it on our Web site at www.SuperSizedKids.com.) Again, it gets them moving.

So go for a walk! And make it fun.

Develop an Obstacle Course

Most kids love creative obstacle courses. If the weather prevents you from making a course outside, make a fun one inside. Use pillows and chairs and blankets and whatever else you need to create tunnels and hurdles and other barriers to get your kids moving. Use your imagination and have fun!

Find a Gym That Has Programs and Equipment for Children

The Deltona YMCA in Orlando, is the first in the country to install KL Hoist exercise equipment, specially designed for safe use by children. "This equipment encourages parents to bring their kids along when they come to work out," says Patti Stephens, wellness coordinator. "Parents can drop their kids off at the front door for a supervised exercise session, then go do their own workout."

The equipment includes both strength training and aerobics. Patti stresses that the staff "mixes things up for the kids so they won't get bored. We'll have them do some strength training, then we'll get them on one of the bikes, then back to strength training." This equipment has proved popular with the Y's after-school program and the home school PE program.

The equipment has a special appeal to kids struggling with their weight, Patti says. A lot of these kids don't participate in sports or other physical activities, whether due to their weight or to lack of skill. But she notes that these kids enjoy some real success on the Hoist equipment—they can do the exercises. And that means they are more likely to stick with it.

We imagine that more and more health clubs and gymnasiums will quickly follow the example of the Deltona YMCA. And even if the gym your family uses doesn't have children's equipment, find out if it offers programs designed for children. Boys and Girls Clubs are an excellent choice. The range of possible activities is limitless, but if you'd like some other ideas, consider these:

- Wake up half an hour earlier and walk the dog through the neighborhood.
- If possible, walk or bike your kids to school.
- Go for a swim together.
- Several evenings a week, plan a fun, outdoor activity for the entire family.

- Consider bike riding, softball, kickball, basketball, hiking, in-line skating, ice skating.
- Get the kids involved in gymnastics, track, football, basketball, lacrosse, swimming, or tennis, or have them take classes in such disciplines as dance, martial arts, ballet, or marching band.
- Meet friends at the playground.
- Park farther out in the lot at a store or mall and walk or skip to the store.
- Walk up steps rather than taking an elevator.

MAKE SURE THE ACTIVITY FITS THE CHILD

Without question, activity benefits every child at every age. But does this mean that every activity is right for every child? No.

Depending on your child's age, he or she may not be ready for certain types of activities. This is especially true when it comes to sports. Children aren't little adults. They go through various developmental stages physically, mentally, and socially.

If your child has expressed an interest in a sport such as soccer or baseball, the American Academy of Pediatrics (AAP) Committee on Sports Medicine and Fitness recommends matching the "demands of the sport or exercise activity to the developmental maturity of the child." In other words, make sure your child is ready physically, mentally, and socially for the skills and demands of that sport; otherwise, what should be a fun experience could turn into frustration.

Consider some general guidelines, recommended by the AAP, that will help you to choose age-appropriate activities for your kids:

- Children aged two to five are beginning to learn the "basics" like throwing, catching, and jumping. Encourage activities that use these skills in noncomplicated ways. (A child this age can catch a ball thrown directly at him but can't catch a ball while running. And the child usually catches with two hands, not one.)

- Children aged six to nine are becoming more accurate in their throwing and kicking. Because their decision-making skills are maturing, they can also handle the basic strategies of simple forms of sports. (If they're playing soccer, for example, they understand that you can kick farther if you rear back; but if they're playing baseball, they would have difficulty knowing when a double play is possible.)

- Children aged ten to twelve are ready for more complex sports. Their ability to learn and understand the strategies required for these sports is growing, and their motor skills are more developed. (They better understand the importance of positioning players and passing required in football and basketball.)

Let's now take a look at several specific sports[9]:

Soccer. The strategies of this sport are difficult for young children to understand. Try versions that allow children to have fun without emphasizing rules. "Beehive" soccer would be one such example (this is where the children "swarm" around the ball without much regard for rules).

Baseball. Because young children are still developing hand-eye coordination, "tee-ball"—in which the ball is placed on a stand rather than pitched—would be appropriate and make the game more enjoyable.

Running/triathlons. These events can be enjoyed by children if the events are specially designed for them. Because children have less tolerance for heat than adults, it is *extremely* important that they remain well hydrated before, during, and after their event. Also make sure that the event emphasizes fun and fitness and not competition.

Skiing. Cross-country skiing can be a great activity for your child. Just be sure to keep the distance appropriate for your child's age. Special downhill skiing equipment has been designed for children as young as three that allows the parent to guide and control movements.

Weight lifting. While children can lift weights, a qualified professional should supervise it—someone who has received training in appropriate techniques for children. Before reaching skeletal maturity (age fifteen for girls and age seventeen for boys), children shouldn't attempt to lift "maximal" weight, the most weight they can lift at one time. Also make sure they avoid movements such as the snatch or the clean and jerk. Power lifting and bodybuilding are *not* recommended.

Whatever sport you and your child choose, keep in mind the goal: to have fun while getting fit.

CLIMB THE ACTIVITY PYRAMID

To end this chapter, we'd like to give you a tool to help you plan an activity schedule for your family.

The activity pyramid on the following page provides you with recommendations for various types of activities and how often your child should engage in them. Take a look at the pyramid and determine if your child is getting enough activity in his or her day.

Did you find any areas of the pyramid where you and your family need some work? That's okay. We have another tool to help, a blank pyramid that you can turn into your family's individual activity pyramid (page 128).

Get your family together and decide what your pyramid will look like. Start at the foundation and list several activities you can do every day as a family. As your activity increases, go to the next level and list those activities that you will do almost every day. Continue up the levels until you are doing activities from the entire pyramid. Remember to choose a variety of enjoyable, age-appropriate activities that your family will continue to do.

And have fun!

The Kids' Activity Pyramid

Get Up, Get Out, Get Fun, and Get Fit with Your Family

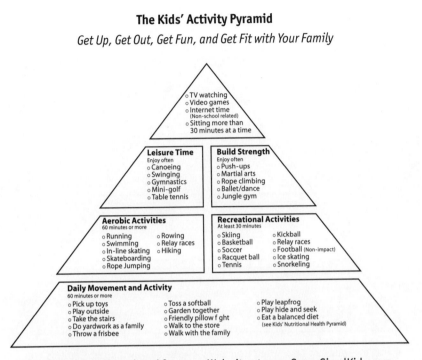

This pyramid can be printed from our Web site at www.SuperSizedKids.com.

Adapted from recommendations by the President's Council on Physical Fitness and the Centers for Disease Control and Prevention.

THE END OF THE STORY

Try to picture Garfield, the ill-tempered cartoon cat. What comes to mind (besides lasagna)? If you know the cartoon, you probably think of him lying down. And what else do you see?

He's a fat feline.

Now switch mental gears and think of a more vintage animated cartoon featuring a blur of a mouse named Speedy Gonzalez—he of the "andale, andale, arriba, arriba, *yeeha!*" tagline. What comes to mind? Probably the cloud of dust he leaves behind each time he takes off running. And what else do you see?

He's one lean rodent.

If you want to gain control over your family's weight, maybe you could learn a thing or two from these celluloid celebrities—and along

The Kids' "Blank" Activity Pyramid

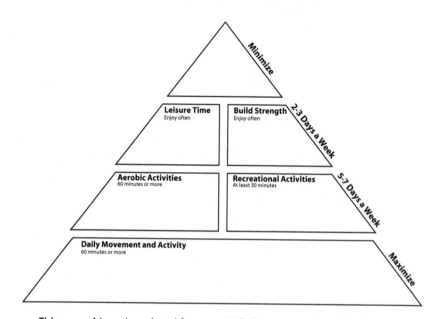

This pyramid can be printed from our Web site at www.SuperSizedKids.com.

with your kids, get off the couch and get moving. Remember, *physical activity* is an indispensable key to keeping those extra pounds at bay.

Bobby sure knows the truth about that. Remember him? He was the boy we met at the beginning of this chapter who wound up dead last every time his class had to run around the school yard.

Well, one day Bobby decided enough was enough. He wouldn't have said it like that, but basically he gave up on Garfield and pursued Speedy. Do you know what he did? One day after he came home from school, he started walking. In a few days he felt good enough to start running. And then he ran. And ran. And ran.

And by the end of the school year, he was coming in first on those school yard runs.

Do you know what else happened? Bobby dropped quite a few pounds, and today, as a young man, he stays at a healthy weight. The increased exercise changed his life; even his eating habits changed. He didn't eat as many desserts or as much junk food as he used to. He just didn't want to.

What caused the change? Bobby didn't want to come in last anymore. And today he wouldn't trade in his new "firsts" for anything.

We don't mean to suggest that your child will move from last to first place in school runs just by getting more active. But we do want to insist that, for our children's sakes, we all need to move exercise from last place on our "to do" lists to something closer to the top.

We wish you could see Bobby's grin. That alone would motivate you.

SIMPLE STEPS THAT WORK

Increase your family's physical activity from minimal to moderate by trying a few of the following activities:

- Shoot some hoops with your child. Kick the soccer ball or throw a baseball in the yard. Or organize a Frisbee football or golf game with the neighborhood children (chances are they, too, need more activity).
- Take walks as a family. Start with short walks of ten or fifteen minutes. (Walks before meals actually reduce a child's appetite.) This can be a great time to talk and interact!
- Take advantage of biking trails in your area. One day each week do this activity as a family. Then if you enjoy it, increase the number of days per week.
- Teach your children to take the stairs instead of the elevator. Or when you take them to the store, park farther out in the parking lot.
- Walk with your children to school.
- Plan a family vacation or weekend trip that involves activity. Hiking, canoeing, kayaking, and biking can all make for great family outings.

- Organize a family contest to see who can be the most active during the day. Have rewards to encourage participation: a favorite CD, an hour at the library reading, a day at the beach.
- Find sports activities you can do as a family. Many churches and community centers sponsor sports that encourage the entire family to participate.

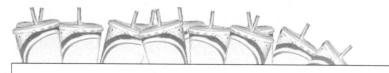

Fifty Ways to SuperSize Your Kids #21

Get some Elmer's and glue your kids to the couch.

9

OVERFED AND UNDERNOURISHED

Food in our country is bountiful, inexpensive, and readily available. And the highly processed foods so unhealthful for us and our children are often the most readily available and the tastiest. Add in the fact that eating is one of life's joys, and it's not hard to see why we've landed in such trouble.

One Harris survey revealed that 84 percent of Americans named eating as their top leisure-time activity![1] It seems that here in the United States, instead of eating to live, we live to eat. And so we've turned ourselves into a nation that loves tasty foods high in "bad" fats and "bad" carbs, low in nutrients, and dense in calories.

Food for Thought

Here in America we may talk healthy, but we eat tasty.

To make things even harder, it's a confusing world out there when it comes to making healthy food choices. Everyone seems to have an opinion about "good" nutrition (and weight loss)—late-night infomercials, diet gurus, the newest kids' cereal, even the local grocery store. All of them broadcast messages about healthful eating.

And yet Americans continue to eat too much of the wrong things.

A federal report released in 2004 found that much of our population is overfed and undernourished.[2] Even though we live in a land of plenty, we aren't making the right food choices and so are coming up short on many nutrients essential to our health.

So what should you put on your table? Let's consider some healthy eating basics that can help control your child's weight, and what you can do to instill these good habits in your children.

GOOD FOOD IS COLORFUL FOOD

First, while your child may struggle with weight issues, it's important to remember that your child is still growing. Many children don't lose a pound, but grow toward a normal BMI as they continue to grow taller. So we always tell parents to focus on healthy eating instead of dieting, a more successful approach in the long run.

Fruits and Vegetables

Did your mother ever tell you to finish your vegetables? Have you heard the maxim that an apple a day keeps the doctor away? Today we recognize both suggestions as wise pieces of advice.

One of the best habits your child can learn is to eat five to seven servings of fruits and vegetables every day. Yet most American kids eat only half the recommended number of servings; they tend to prefer salty, sugary, fatty foods instead.

What's so special about fruits and vegetables? They are low in calories and high in fiber, two very healthy benefits, especially for children struggling with their weight, as fiber provides a feeling of satisfaction when consumed. In fact, surveys have found that Americans who eat the most fruits and vegetables are the least likely to be overweight.[3] Fruits and vegetables are loaded with the vitamins and minerals your child needs for growth, and they also contain beneficial compounds known as phytochemicals.

Phytochemicals (which we like to call fighter chemicals) act like soldiers: They protect you and your children against disease. Some battle heart disease, others blunt cancer, and still others promote healthy immune systems. Daily consumption of fruits and vegetables not only reduces the risk of these diseases but also helps in weight control.

Offer many colors of fruits and vegetables, since each color has its own phytochemicals:

- Try "sunshine yellows" like grapefruit, squash, yellow peppers, and pineapple.
- Feed them "bright oranges" such as cantaloupe, carrots, sweet potatoes, and oranges.
- Serve "fire engine reds" like strawberries, tomatoes, red peppers, and raspberries.
- Dish up the "blues" with blueberries, eggplant, purple cabbage, and plums.
- Put a little "green" on your plate like spinach, kiwifruit, edamame (bright green soybeans still in the pod), and honeydew melon.
- And don't forget the "whites and browns" like cauliflower, bananas, mushrooms, and brown pears.

Don't let beige foods—such as pasta, white rice, and mashed potatoes—dominate your child's plate. Instead, for the best nutrition possible, make sure you offer two or three deep, rich colors at each meal.

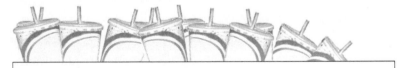

Fifty Ways to SuperSize Your Kids   #22

Ignore fruits and vegetables in your children's diet.

And how can you get in five to seven servings each day? Consider a few tips:

- Add fruit to your child's cereal at breakfast.
- Pour a small glass of 100 percent fruit juice to drink with breakfast or with a snack.
- Put vegetables on pizza and sandwiches, in spaghetti sauce, even add shredded vegetables to your favorite meat loaf recipe.
- A piece of fresh fruit or a small homemade fruit smoothie makes a healthy dessert.
- Offer snacks of fruits and vegetables instead of the typical high-fat, high-sugar, high-salt ones.
- Don't forget vegetable-based soups and salads.

Serving sizes will vary depending on the age of your child (see the next chapter), but the important thing is to make sure your child eats fruits and vegetables throughout the day.

Protein

Your child's body uses protein to build, repair, and maintain tissues, especially during their years of childhood growth. Protein foods also help your child feel more satisfied after a meal and keep him or her from feeling hungry again too soon.

Proteins are found in many foods, such as meats, poultry, eggs, and fish. These also provide iron, B vitamins, and some minerals, but they can be high in saturated fats, cholesterol, and calories. So bake, broil, grill, or stir-fry these foods. We now know that plant sources of protein are just as healthy as animal sources—and in some cases, much more so. These include legumes (dried beans and peas), nuts and seeds, and soy products. Plant proteins are naturally low in saturated fats, contain no cholesterol, and have the added benefit of being high in fiber and phytochemicals.

In addition, the latest research shows that a boiled or scrambled egg or two a day is not bad for your child's heart and health—as long as you use an oil high in monounsaturated fat to cook the egg (see "Fat Facts" later in this chapter). In fact, egg yolks contain two powerful phytochemicals (lutein and zeaxanthin) that promote eye health.

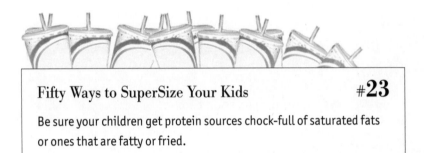

Fifty Ways to SuperSize Your Kids   #**23**

Be sure your children get protein sources chock-full of saturated fats or ones that are fatty or fried.

Depending on your child's age, he or she will need two to three protein servings daily (equal to four to six ounces). Consider a few ideas for getting enough protein in your child's meals:

- Boiled egg at breakfast
- Small handful of chopped walnuts on oatmeal
- Turkey sandwich or low-fat bean burrito for lunch
- Chicken breast and tofu stir-fry at dinner
- Peanut butter (choose "natural" brands that contain no "bad" fats)
- A small handful of nuts or seeds as a snack

Whole Grains

Has anyone told you that carbohydrates (starches, grains) are bad for you and that eating them will lead to weight gain? If so, you might feel hesitant to feed your child anything starchy.

But carbohydrates provide fuel for our bodies. They provide your child with the energy to breathe, walk, play, and even do schoolwork.

The truth is, good carbohydrates should be the foundation of a healthy diet. Not only do they provide energy, they also provide vitamins and minerals, are a wonderful source of fiber, and contain phytochemicals. The problem is that we eat too many bad carbohydrates stripped of these health-promoting properties.

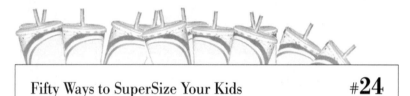

Fifty Ways to SuperSize Your Kids   #24

Feed your kids plenty of highly processed, sugar-laden food.

"Bad" carbohydrates include simple or processed sugars—soft drinks, candy, sweet snack foods—and highly refined starches: white rice, white bread, potatoes without the skin, most cereals, most pastas, and most baked goods. These foods contain little or no fiber at all. But fiber works in several ways to help with weight control. Eating high-fiber foods gives a sense of fullness, which can help to control how much one eats. In addition, high-fiber foods take longer to leave the stomach, which delays a sense of hunger. Highly refined, processed foods have lost most of their fiber and so provide a concentrated source of calories. Because we don't feel as full and get hungry sooner after we eat "bad" carbohydrates, it becomes easier to snack between meals and get more calories than we need. These extra calories, more likely than not, will be stored as fat and can lead to weight gain.

Here's an example of how eating low fiber (highly processed) versus high fiber (whole or unprocessed) works in real life. Suppose your child eats a sugar-coated, highly processed cereal soaked in high-fat milk for breakfast, along with a low-fiber, high-sugar Pop-Tart. Chances are he will feel hungry again in only a few hours. If he's at school, he'll probably buy something from a vending machine—and

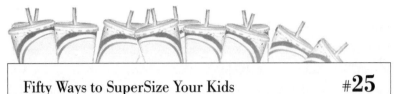

Fifty Ways to SuperSize Your Kids   **#25**

Give your kids several servings each day of highly refined starches, such as white rice, white bread, potatoes without the skin, pasta, and baked goods.

very few vending machines have healthy food for children. How much better if your child had a whole grain, low-sugar dry cereal or bowl of oatmeal, along with a favorite fruit and nonfat or skim milk. Add a small handful of nuts, and he would sail right through to lunch without needing to hit the vending machines.

Remember that highly refined carbohydrates have almost all of their fiber, vitamins and minerals, and phytochemicals removed. What's left? Calories without benefits. While you can let your child partake of these foods sparingly, the less the better.

Children need six to nine grain foods daily of varying serving sizes, depending on their age (see chart on page 165). A worthwhile goal is to have at least half, or no fewer than three, of your child's grain servings consist of whole grain foods (and more is better!). Research shows that eating whole grains can protect against heart disease by lowering cholesterol levels, reduce the risk for certain cancers, and possibly even help to protect against type 2 diabetes.

To make sure that your child gets a whole grain, read the ingredients list. The grain (wheat, rice, corn, oats, etc.) should be first on the list and the words "whole" or "whole grain" should also appear before the grain's name. And don't be afraid to try a new whole grain! Millet, couscous, quinoa, wheat berries, etc., can all add a new flavor and texture to your meals. You can find them at most grocery stores and health food stores.

You may have heard that "stone ground" grains are healthier than other types. It's important to read the ingredients list, however, because products labeled "stone ground," "multigrain," "100 percent wheat," or "bran" may actually contain little or no whole grain. And don't be swayed by the color of a processed food. Don't be fooled, for example, by the word "unbleached": It means only that the refined flour is still yellow because it hasn't been bleached yet—so this type of flour may not be a whole grain and would be a less healthy choice. "Brown" bread is often brown because of molasses, not because it's made from a whole grain. Again, look for the words "whole" or "whole grain" before the name of the grain.

Consider a few ideas for getting more whole grains in your kids' diet:

- Whole grain toast or sandwich bread
- Whole grain waffles
- Whole grain dry cereal; oatmeal or other whole grain hot cereal
- Whole grain crackers with soup
- Whole grain tortilla burrito (corn or wheat) for lunch or a snack
- Brown rice and stir-fry vegetables
- Brown rice and beans
- Whole grain quinoa side dish for dinner

We should warn you, too, that cereal companies have begun to produce "whole grain" cereals. Some of these cereals, however, are very high in added sugar. Don't rely on the advertising; look at the label to see what you're really getting. A good rule of thumb: Look for a cereal that contains less than six grams of sugar per serving (this will be listed as "Sugars" under "Total Carbohydrate").

Dairy Products

A recent study found that Americans are consuming 38 percent fewer calories from milk than they did in 1977. The biggest drop in milk consumption occurred in two- through eighteen-year-olds[4]—yet these are crucial years for growing a child's bones, teeth, and muscles.

More and more researchers believe, as we do, that it is not necessary to rely solely on dairy foods for calcium or protein once a child reaches age three or four. According to research by Katherine Tucker of Tufts University, if we focus more on whole foods, such as whole grains, legumes, and produce, we will create a positive mineral balance that can meet our children's daily calcium needs. Other good sources of calcium are nonfat yogurt, calcium-fortified soy products, and calcium-fortified orange juice. Still, most children and adults do not get enough calcium without consuming nonfat milk and/or calcium supplements.

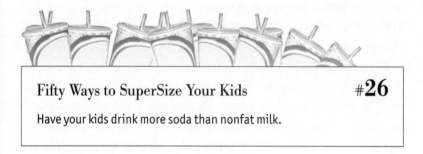

Fifty Ways to SuperSize Your Kids   **#26**

Have your kids drink more soda than nonfat milk.

Despite our ability to easily meet our children's calcium needs, the American Academy of Pediatrics warns that children and adolescents in the United States are not getting enough calcium. Because of this deficiency, the academy recommends a daily diet that includes:

- Fat-free milk
- Fat-free yogurt
- Low-fat cheese
- Other calcium-rich foods such as tofu (processed with calcium), calcium-fortified soy or rice milk, calcium-fortified orange juice and dry cereals, turnip greens, dried figs, okra, oranges, broccoli, and pinto beans

Food for Thought

One cup of whole milk has as much artery-clogging saturated fat as one hot dog, five strips of bacon, a Snickers candy bar, or a fast-food hamburger.[5]

If your family is hooked on whole milk, make the transition to skim milk gradually. Walt's wife, Barb, started with 2 percent milk; the initial complaining soon died down. About a month later she began purchasing 1 percent milk. That transition went over okay, but she knew skim milk would be a tougher sell. So after another month Barb started mixing 1 percent and skim. After a few more months she made the final transition to skim milk. (Barb was a bit sneaky about this. She kept the lower-fat milk in the full-fat milk container—and the kids never knew!)

Children and adolescents who cannot or will not consume dairy products should consider the use of a mineral supplement. If your child takes a calcium supplement, be sure that the dose is taken with food at two meals, at the least. Calcium is better absorbed with food, and our bodies cannot absorb a whole day's dose at one time. It is also important to get adequate amounts of vitamin D, either by taking a supplement or by enjoying sunlight.

The National Dairy Council has found that the average teenager drinks only one glass of milk a day, but twice as many sodas.[6] They say children need two to three servings of dairy foods daily. Focus on nonfat dairy products and other calcium-rich foods. Nonfat dairy products (compared to those with fat) are lower in calories, but still provide the needed amounts of protein, calcium, vitamin D, and other essential nutrients.

If your child is lactose intolerant, you can purchase dairy products or supplements that contain the lactase enzyme (like Lactaid). Or try yogurt or hard cheeses. Remember that white cheeses are normally much lower in saturated fat than yellow cheeses. Or look for low-fat varieties. Cheeses are naturally low in lactose, and most of us can enjoy these without any problem. Calcium-fortified dairy substitutes, such as soy milk and rice milk, can also fill this gap. When using a dairy substitute, choose a brand that offers the same amount of calcium and protein as cow's milk and is also fortified with vitamins D and B_{12}. You may also want to meet with a registered dietitian to ensure that your child is getting the nutrients found in milk.

One caution: Everyone and their brother is trying to get flavored milk drinks into our schools. Even the chocolate manufacturer Cadbury has begun making milk drinks—strawberry, kiwi, and banana. Is it still milk? Sure—but these versions have a lot of extra calories, due to all the sweeteners added. So don't consider them pure milk!

Can drinking nonsweetened milk help your child lose weight? Researchers are busy studying this question. A small number of studies have found that adults who include low-fat dairy products in their reduced-calorie eating plan have lost weight. Why? It may be that calcium helps your body burn fat at a faster rate.[7] And some 2001 research reported that dairy foods might help children maintain their body-fat levels. Not all health experts, however, agree on the role dairy plays (if any) in weight loss, and at least one study has found that dairy products did not aid in weight loss.

Consider a few ways to include calcium-rich foods in your child's eating plan:

- A glass of fat-free (skim) milk or calcium-fortified orange juice at breakfast
- A slice of low-fat cheese on a sandwich for lunch or with whole grain crackers for snacks
- Pinto beans and brown rice for lunch
- Vegetable stir-fry that includes broccoli and tofu for dinner
- A carton of low-fat or nonfat yogurt for dessert at dinner—and it's even better if mixed with fresh fruit

Fat Facts

For the past several decades health experts have been warning us not to eat too much fat. High-fat diets have been linked to heart disease, many cancers, diabetes, and obesity.

When you visit your local bookstore, you see low-fat cookbooks lining the shelves. The food industry has created hundreds, if not thousands, of low-fat or no-fat products—and products that *never had* fat advertise "fat-free" on their labels. Fat seems to be on everyone's mind.

Do you know that we actually need certain fats to remain healthy? This is especially true for growing children. Some necessary fats transport nutrients between our cells and store energy for later use. And fat contributes to a feeling of fullness and helps us not to be hungry again too soon. The problem is not fat per se, but that we are eating too many of the unhealthful fats and not enough of the healthful ones.

The concern with eating too many unhealthful fats is that these tend to make our total cholesterol and LDL ("bad" or "lethal") cholesterol go up. This type of cholesterol can form deposits on artery walls, causing blockages that may lead to heart disease and heart attacks. Replacing the unhealthful fats with healthful fats helps to bring our total cholesterol and LDL cholesterol levels down and may even increase our levels of HDL ("good" or "healthy") cholesterol. HDL cholesterol acts like a garbage truck, carrying "bad" cholesterol to the liver, where it gets broken down and excreted. Let's take a closer look at several of the fats:

Saturated fats. We classify these as "bad" or unhealthful fats. They come mainly from animal foods, such as meat, poultry, and milk that is not skim (fat-free). They usually remain solid at room temperature. They trigger the liver to produce more cholesterol and LDL ("bad") cholesterol, which, when too high, is linked to heart disease. Children simply *do not need* saturated fat in their diets.

Unsaturated fats. There are two types of unsaturated fats: *monounsaturated* and *polyunsaturated*. The former we consider

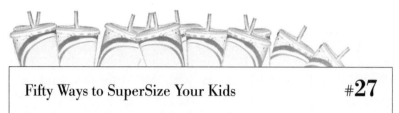

Fifty Ways to SuperSize Your Kids   **#27**

Insist that your kids eat or drink full-fat dairy products.

"good" or healthful fat; the latter is more of a mixed bag. Monounsaturated fats trigger less production of cholesterol and LDL ("bad" or "lethal") cholesterol, and more HDL ("good" or "healthy") cholesterol. Canola oil, olive oil, and nuts are great sources of this fat. Polyunsaturated fats trigger lower cholesterol and LDL cholesterol, but also less HDL cholesterol. This fat is found in corn, soybean, and sunflower oils and in seafood. Unsaturated fats tend to remain liquid at room temperature.

Omega-3 fatty acids. These fats have been receiving a lot of attention lately. They are highly polyunsaturated fats that reduce blood clotting and protect against hardening of the arteries. They are found in fatty fish (tuna and salmon), as well as nuts, flaxseed, and canola oil.

Omega-6 fatty acids. These are another category of polyunsaturated fats. They are found in corn, cottonseed, sunflower, and safflower oils, as well as some soy products. Americans tend to consume these in higher amounts than recommended. They may offer some protection against heart disease, but may also lower HDL ("good") cholesterol. Use them in moderation, concentrating on increasing your intake of omega-3s.

Trans-fatty acids. When it comes to fat, this is the new bad boy on the block. We've known about these fats, also called trans fats, since the 1960s, but recently have begun to learn how they negatively impact our health. While trans-fatty acids are found naturally in some foods, the majority are man-made, formed during the process of hydrogenation (taking a liquid fat and making it more solid).

Trans fats act like saturated fats in the bloodstream and can raise cholesterol levels. As we'll discuss in Chapter 13, "Battle of the Bulge on the Statehouse Steps," we believe that all food labels should indicate whether the product contains trans fats. In the meantime, you can identify them by looking for the term "hydrogenated" on the label (usually in very small print). Trans-fatty acids are a health risk for children and should be eliminated from their diets or at least limited as much as possible.

Foods that typically contain trans-fatty acids are stick margarine, vegetable shortening, some peanut butters, prepared cakes, cookies, crackers, snack foods, fried fast foods, and other commercially fried foods.

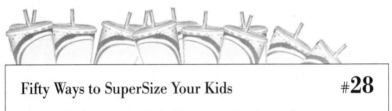

Fifty Ways to SuperSize Your Kids   #28

Give your kids snacks loaded with saturated and trans fats.

Fat is important to the taste and texture of many enjoyable foods, and trying to eliminate all fat would be impossible (and not very tasty). It would also harm our health. We shouldn't go overboard and cut back too much on fat. Children under the age of two need full-fat products. Their brains are still "under construction" and need fat to develop normally. After the age of two the key is moderation and focusing on healthy fats while reducing or eliminating the "bad" or undesirable fats.

Monitor the type of fat you are using. If you find that your family is eating a large amount of saturated (mainly animal) fat, consider a few tips for more healthful fat habits:

- Center meals around plant proteins, such as pinto beans, black beans, and soy products.
- Use more lean meat, poultry, seafood, and nonfat dairy products.

- Cut back on or eliminate the amount of fried foods your family eats.
- Switch to an oil higher in monounsaturated fats, such as olive or canola oil.
- Begin to enjoy small servings of nuts.

The "Less Is Better" Foods

Face it: Children (and most adults) would prefer to make salty, sugary, fatty foods the mainstay of their diets. These foods provide little in the way of nutrition, however, and a lot in the way of calories.

Teach your children that these foods (chips, candy, cookies, etc.) can be enjoyed occasionally (and we stress *occasionally*). Focus instead on foods that provide what the body needs for good health: fruits and vegetables, whole grains, nonfat dairy products, lean meats, poultry and seafood, and nuts and seeds.

ARE YOU LABEL SAVVY?

Making wise food choices helps your child move toward a healthy weight—and food labels can provide you with information to make these choices. The nutrition label shows the amount of various food components *in one serving* of the product. Here's what to look at:

1. The serving size, which appears immediately below "Nutrition Facts," tells you how much of the product is in one serving. This will guide you to know how much to serve of this food (you may find that you have been eating two or three servings of this food—and more calories—when you thought you were eating only one).

2. Pay attention to the "Calories." This lets you know how many total calories are in a serving so you can decide how much of this food to eat and how often. Calories from fat are also listed here, but for weight loss the total calories, rather than fat calories, are more important.

3. The amounts of "Total Fat" (the more healthful choices have higher unsaturated fats than saturated fats), "Cholesterol," "Sodium," and "Sugars," although important for *all* children, are critical if your child has elevated cholesterol, high blood pressure, or diabetes. Check with your physician to determine the amounts considered healthful.

4. If you are concerned about certain nutrients, check out the "% Daily Value." This lets you know if there is a little or a lot of something in one serving of this food. Here's a good rule of thumb: 5 percent DV or less of a nutrient is low, and 20 percent DV or more of a nutrient is high. (An example: A food that lists the % DV of calcium at 5 percent would not be a good source of calcium, since it provides only 5 percent of an adult's recommended daily intake.)

Paying attention to what is on the label doesn't mean that you have to stop eating a food because it's too high in calories. It does mean that you will make informed decisions about the foods you eat and can adjust serving sizes and balance higher-calorie foods with lower-calorie foods.

BEWARE THE LIQUID CALORIES

We have to hand it to the advertisers—when thirsty children sit down to eat with their friends, they almost always reach for a soft drink. Kids today drink twice as many sodas as they did in the late 1970s, according to the American Institute for Cancer Research. This concerns us for two reasons. First, a growing body of evidence suggests that obesity in children may be related to the amount of soft drinks they consume. Second, when children drink more sodas, their intake of healthy beverages, such as nonfat milk and water, decreases, along with their nutrient intake.

Soda is also loaded with caffeine, which can cause nervousness, irritability, restlessness, and fidgetiness in children. No doubt healthier liquids lack a kick like Mountain Dew, Surge, or Jolt, all of which deliver a powerful caffeine punch, but some soft drinks also have over ninety milligrams of caffeine per twenty ounces—the equivalent of a five-ounce cup of brewed coffee.

Realize, too, that fruit juice has as many calories as soda; therefore, water really needs to become the liquid of choice. Your children should get their calories from whole fruits, such as oranges, apples, tangerines, and grapefruit.

If you want to give them a fruit beverage, look for products labeled as "fruit juice" and avoid "fruit drinks." To be labeled as a fruit juice, the Food and Drug Administration mandates that a product be 100 percent fruit juice. Any beverage less than 100 percent fruit juice must be described as a "drink," "beverage," or "cocktail." In general, fruit drinks add sweeteners and may contribute to SuperSizing kids. One study found a link between fruit drink intake in excess of twelve ounces per day and obesity.[8] Fruit drinks also tend to contain large amounts of high-fructose corn syrup, a type of sugar that appears to switch off the sensation of fullness as we eat, so the more sugary drinks we drink, the more we *want* to drink.

Remember, just eight ounces a day of a sugary drink leads to an extra six pounds a year. A twelve-ounce can of soda has 150 calories; so one a day leads to about ten extra pounds a year. And if your kids are drinking a twenty-ounce regular soda, that's *250* calories, which almost doubles the weight they could gain. Unfortunately, in our experience it's not unusual for a child to drink a six-pack of soda a day, which adds about 1,000 extra calories. We just *have* to wean our kids off of soda and sugary fruit drinks!

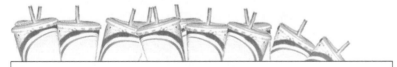

Fifty Ways to SuperSize Your Kids	#29
Choose fruit drinks instead of 100 percent fruit juice for your child.	

Walt remembers when his daughter, Kate, went soda-free. The overwhelming sweetness of the first soda she drank after she had given it up just stunned her. Her little lip wrinkled up, and she snorted, "This is so sweet! What *is* this?"

"It's Coke, honey."

"Is it a new one?"

"No, it's the regular stuff."

To help wean your kids off the sugar water, try switching at first to C2 or Pepsi Edge, then maybe to the eight-ounce can. Perhaps the next step is carbonated or noncarbonated mineral water. And eventually get them to the point where their beverage of choice is water. That could take some time, but it will be well worth it.

It's also important to drink lots of water, ideally eight servings of eight ounces a day. Water plays an essential role in maintaining health by regulating body temperature; carrying nutrients and oxygen to cells; cushioning joints; protecting organs and tissues; removing toxins; and maintaining strength and endurance. And children need *more* water per pound of body weight than adults, for the simple reason that their bodies are still growing and demanding the hydration found in plain water. Fluids in the blood transport glucose to the muscles and carry away lactic acid. Fluids in urine eliminate waste products from the body. Fluids in sweat dissipate excess heat and cool the body.

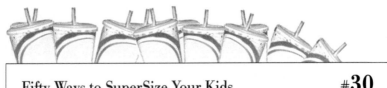

Fifty Ways to SuperSize Your Kids   #**30**

Encourage your kids to drink anything but water.

Only use sources of fluids other than water in appropriate amounts. While sports drinks such as Gatorade and Allsports, 100 percent fruit juices, and nonfat milk all contain water, they also deliver additional calories. If your child plays a sport for an extended period, sports drinks may be appropriate. They contain water, with minimal glucose or sugar, and a touch of electrolytes (primarily sodium and potassium) and help to keep young bodies hydrated.

Finally, don't think you're off the hook, parents. An American Dietetic Association survey found that the biggest influence on the amount of sugared drinks consumed by children was—you guessed it—their parents. So take that small step with your child and work together to drink fewer sugared drinks.

Remember, you really can't improve on fresh, cool water. Drinking water is habit-forming, so help your children gain this healthy, lifetime habit.

HEALTHY EATING IN A NUTSHELL

Healthy eating is balanced eating, based on making informed choices. To start down the road of healthy eating, make sure that your child eats a balance of needed nutrients throughout the day. Consider a few tips from the American Dietetic Association:

- Half of your child's calories, or even a little more, should come from "good" carbohydrate sources, such as fruits, vegetables, and whole grains. Limit refined, highly processed carbohydrates.
- Your child's protein needs will vary depending on age and whether he or she is going through a growth phase. Including a quality protein source at each meal and snack will ensure adequate intake. And don't forget to include plant proteins!
- Fat is essential for children under the age of two and should account for 30 to 40 percent of total calories. After this, the amount of saturated fat in the diet can be dramatically decreased or even eliminated. Focus on healthful fats like those found in canola oil, olive oil, nuts, and seeds.

- Added sugars should only be a very small part of your child's diet, making up no more than 25 percent of his or her daily calorie intake—the lower the better.
- Don't neglect the fiber. Children one to three years old need 19 grams a day; four- to eight-year-olds need 25 grams a day; boys nine to thirteen need 31 grams a day, and girls nine to thirteen need 26 grams a day.[9] Fiber also helps with weight control. Not only does fiber help us feel full sooner, most high-fiber foods are lower in calories.

FAST FOOD EQUALS FAST WEIGHT GAIN

With all the demands on our time, it's no wonder that processed foods have become so popular. After all, they are quick and easy to fix. The downside is they're usually loaded with empty calories and stripped of most nutrients. So how can you start using more "whole" foods and fewer processed foods?

Gradually make the change from highly processed foods to whole foods. Sherri's husband, George, loves beans and rice. One day she decided to switch to brown rice. While George didn't feel terribly excited about the change, he went along with it. The next time, she served white rice. She kept alternating, and after a month or two George admitted that he actually preferred the taste of brown rice—something that surprised him. And it's been brown rice ever since.

Another big time-saver in our hectic lives is fast food. You probably can't ban your kids from fast-food restaurants, but you can certainly cut back considerably. Further, you can teach your children how to order smarter, because fast-food chains are scrambling to offer more healthful items. But be careful! Items that you think are more healthful might not be.

- Watch the salad dressing. Regular ranch dressing can supply up to a whopping 20 percent of a child's daily fat needs in one serving. Go for low-calorie or no-calorie dressing. Look for dressings with olive oil or other good oils. Or use only one-fourth to one-half of the dressing packet.

- Some fast-food salads contain more calories and fat grams than burgers. A taco salad at Taco Bell has 380 calories and forty-two fat grams, and the greens and tomatoes arrive in a fried flour taco shell! If this is your favorite fast-food item, don't eat the shell or order the salad without it.

- If you're looking for healthier alternatives, consider pita sandwiches and broiled chicken sandwiches. Quizno's, Subway, and Schlotzsky's Deli have all stepped up with chicken and turkey sandwiches that average six grams of fat or less per serving. Even better, Quizno's, Jason's Deli, Fazoli's, Au Bon Pain, and Ruby Tuesday are eliminating trans fat from all or most items on their menus. Pita sandwiches are making headway as well. And don't forget to ask what whole grain bread choices are available. To reduce fat and calories even more, leave off the cheese and mayo and go with mustard. Don't be afraid to ask for extra lettuce and tomatoes.

- On those occasions when you do order a hamburger, go for the single burger only, or a veggie burger, with no cheese.

- Teach your children that items with chicken or fish will usually contain less fat and fewer calories than the beef or pork versions. Pizzas dotted with pieces of chicken have roughly half the fat of a pepperoni or sausage version.

- Beware of "crispy" chicken sandwiches, fried fish sandwiches, or Original Recipe chicken at KFC. These contain considerably more fat grams than baked or broiled chicken; they contain even more fat than a single patty hamburger. The crispy chicken might be finger-lickin' good, but as the saying goes, "Put it on the lips, wear it on the hips!"

AN OLD PYRAMID GETS A MAKEOVER

In 1992 the USDA developed a Food Guide Pyramid as an easy-to-follow schematic to healthy eating. For the last four years food scientists, physicians, health experts, and policy gurus throughout the country, at the USDA and at the Department of Health and Human Services, have reevaluated this pyramid and in January 2005 published a brand new set of Dietary Guidelines for Americans (you can find them at www.SuperSizedKids.com).

In April of 2005, the USDA shocked the nutritional world by not proposing a replacement pyramid but recommending twelve replacement pyramids!

And you know what? We think they did a pretty good job.

The USDA took the thirteen-year-old food pyramid, turned it on its side, and added a staircase for exercise. Called "MyPyramid," the new graphics place the food groups as rainbow-colored bands running vertically from the tip to the base. The black-and-white illustration that follows gives you an idea of what the new pyramid looks like; on the Web site (you can find the MyPyramid system at www.SuperSizedKids.com) the colors appear as follows, from left to right: orange for grains, green for vegetables, red for fruits, a yellow sliver for oils, blue for dairy products, and purple for meats and beans. Preferred foods such as grains, vegetables, fruits, and nonfat dairy products have wider bands.

MyPyramid works best by accessing the system through the Internet in order to get customized personal recommendations on the daily calorie needs for each family member based on the 2005 Dietary Guidelines.

MyPyramid also allows parents to find up-to-date food guidance and suggestions for making smart choices from each food group. For those who do not have Internet access at home, the MyPyramid programs will be available through computers at public libraries, health departments, and school libraries. Here's a summary of some of the major features of MyPyramid:

MyPyramid

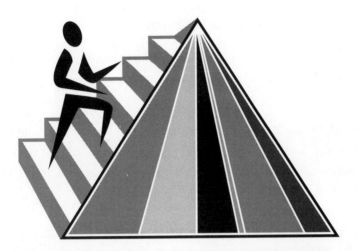

Courtesy of the United States Department of Agriculture.

- **Personalization:** The kinds and amounts of food to eat each day are personalized for you based upon your sex, weight, and daily activity.
- **Gradual improvement:** Encouraged by the slogan "Steps to a Healthier You," we can all benefit from taking small steps to improve our diet and lifestyle each day.
- **Physical activity:** The steps and the person climbing them (as pictured above), serve as a reminder of the importance of daily physical activity.
- **Variety of foods:** The six color bands in MyPyramid represent the five food groups and oils. Nutritious foods from all groups are needed each day for good health.
- **Moderation:** The narrowing of each food group from bottom to top represents moderation. The wider base stands for foods with little or no saturated fats, added sugars, or caloric sweeteners.
- **Proportionality:** The different widths of the food group bands suggest how much food a person should choose from each

group. The widths are just a general guide, not exact proportions. You'll have to check the MyPyramid computer program for the amounts that are right for you and each of your children.

The new food guidance system utilizes a variety of interactive technologies found at the MyPyramid Web site. Here are just a few of the features:

- **MyPyramid Plan:** Obtain a quick estimate of what and how much food you and each of your children should eat from the different food groups by entering your age, gender, and activity level.
- **MyPyramid Tracker:** Get more detailed information on your diet quality and physical activity status by comparing a day's worth of foods eaten with current nutrition guidance. Relevant nutrition and physical activity messages are tailored to your desire to maintain your current weight or to lose weight.
- **Inside MyPyramid:** Get in-depth information for every food group, including recommended daily amounts in commonly used measures, like cups and ounces, with examples and everyday tips. The section also includes recommendations for choosing healthy oils, discretionary calories, and physical activity.
- **Start Today:** Obtain tips and resources that include downloadable suggestions on all the food groups and physical activity, as well as a worksheet to track what you are eating.

We were happy to learn that the USDA plans many future enhancements to MyPyramid, including features that make it possible for parents to make specific food choices by group, look at everyday portions of favorite foods, and adjust their choices to meet their and their children's daily needs.

Even better, the USDA plans a child-friendly version of MyPyramid for teachers and children ages six to eleven years old, with healthy messages about the importance of making smart eating and physical activity choices. As this information comes on line, we'll have it all at www.SuperSizedKids.com.

Dr. Larimore reviewed the studies considered by the USDA in coming up with their new pyramids when he developed his own food pyramid for children and teens, which was first published in the book *The Highly Healthy Child*. The advantage of this pyramid over the newer USDA pyramids is that it is accessible without a computer and the Internet, it is simple and easy to understand, and it clearly shows you the most healthy foods in the larger base sections and the least healthy foods at the top.

Consider the following building blocks of nutritional health that should help you encourage a lifetime of good eating habits for your child (page 156). Don't forget: The lower levels of the pyramid are the most important!

PLANNING YOUR FAMILY'S FOOD PYRAMID

On page 157 we've provided a blank food pyramid to help review and improve your child's meals over the next two weeks. If you would like to track your progress week by week, more blank pyramids can be printed from our Web site at www.SuperSizedKids.com, or you can make photocopies of these pyramids before you fill them out.

In one blank pyramid make a mark for every serving at each meal during the next week. Then compare your child's experience with the ideal pyramid above.

As you study your results, what nutritional adjustments could you most easily make? What simple steps could you take to begin improving your or your child's food pyramid? Using a second blank pyramid, plan your family's meals for the next week. And remember, you don't have to change everything at once. Pick a simple step or two and take it. And have fun!

SIMPLE STEPS THAT WORK

There are a lot of little steps you can use to improve nutrition. Try as many as you'd like. You might be surprised how easy it is for you and your child to start eating your way to better health (see page 158).

Dr. Walt's Food Pyramid for Children and Teens

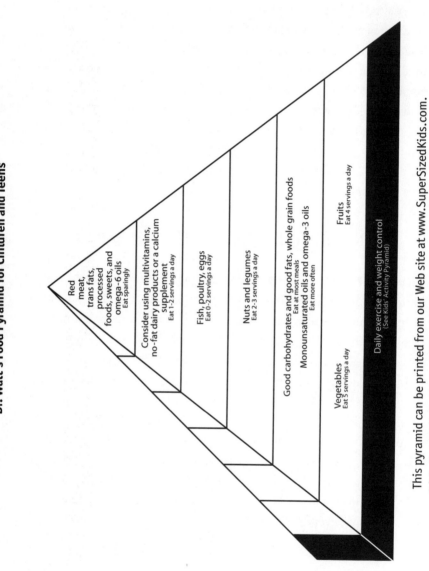

Red meat, trans fats, processed foods, sweets, and omega-6 oils
Eat sparingly

Consider using multivitamins, no-fat dairy products or a calcium supplement
Eat 1-2 servings a day

Fish, poultry, eggs
Eat 0-2 servings a day

Nuts and legumes
Eat 2-3 servings a day

Good carbohydrates and good fats, whole grain foods
Eat at most meals
Monounsaturated oils and omega-3 oils
Eat more often

Vegetables
Eat 5 servings a day

Fruits
Eat 4 servings a day

Daily exercise and weight control
(See Kids' Activity Pyramid)

This pyramid can be printed from our Web site at www.SuperSizedKids.com.

Originally published in *The Highly Healthy Child*, by W. L. Larimore, A. Sorenson, and S. Sorenson (Grand Rapids, MI: Zondervan Publishers, 2004). Used with permission.

The Kids' "Blank" Food Pyramid

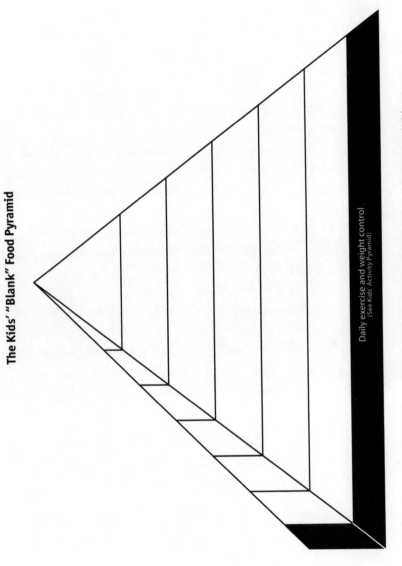

Daily exercise and weight control
(See Kids' Activity Pyramid)

This pyramid can be printed from our Web site at www.SuperSizedKids.com.

- Avoid sugar-laden soft drinks and fruit drinks. Instead, drink water, and then drink some more water.
- If your tap water tastes bad or you fear contamination, filter it.
- Keep a pitcher of water in the refrigerator so it's cold and inviting.
- If your child is drinking twenty ounces or more of soft drinks daily, start to cut back by switching to twelve-ounce cans. Once this takes hold, cut back to eight ounces. Eventually cut back to having soft drinks only very rarely, with water becoming the beverage of choice.
- Switch to a low-sugar drink or sugar-free drink. Alternate between this and water until your child develops a taste for water.
- Serve sugared drinks in a small glass with ice, increasing the amount of ice and decreasing the amount of beverage.
- Don't forget that fruits and vegetables are chock-full of water!
- Start buying whole grain bread; try whole grain pastas (which can be very tasty).
- Add whole grain barley or brown rice to soup.
- When you feel you have to have some fast food, decline the offer to supersize your order.
- When looking for a quick lunch, don't overlook the humble baked potato. Be sure the toppings are healthful, and you have a great choice to go with your side salad.

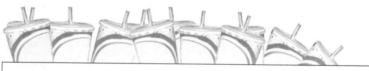

Fifty Ways to SuperSize Your Kids   #31

Feed your kids crispy chicken or fried foods.

10

GEARING UP FOR HEALTHY FAMILY MEALS

Not too long ago, Sherri met with Anne and her daughter, Heather. They had come to her office after Heather confessed that some of her classmates had made snide comments about her weight. Anne thought it might help to meet with a registered dietitian to get some counsel in changing the family's eating habits.

The trio talked about a typical day for Heather—her school activities, what she liked to eat, her TV habits, whether she played outside. Sherri also asked if the family had any habits that fostered good health. Anne cleared her throat and admitted, "Well, we really don't do anything healthy together."

Sherri went over some basic ideas for healthy eating and stressed the importance of getting in some good, appropriate activity. She also asked Heather what she thought she could do to get healthier. She came up with several ideas, and they put together a plan to meet these goals. Mother and daughter both saw the plan as doable and committed the whole family to work on it.

A week later Sherri received a phone call from Anne. Things weren't working out so well; would she mind sending a menu? Sherri put together some suggestions for meals and dropped them in the mail.

Sometime later Sherri ran into Anne at a local mall. They talked for a bit, and then Sherri asked how Heather was doing. Anne sighed and confessed that she had given up trying to help her daughter lose weight. She had simply grown tired of hearing Heather whine about no chips in the house.

Unfortunately Sherri sees the same story repeated with many other clients. Parents want to do what's best for their children, but all too often their good intentions fall by the wayside at the first hint of resistance.

YOU MAKE THE CHOICES

Many sources influence your child's food choices: friends, media, even school. But after what you've already read, it shouldn't surprise you to learn that *you* play the biggest role in the food choices your child makes.

Nearly four years ago the American Dietetic Association Foundation surveyed parents and children to determine what they saw as the biggest influences on children's weight, eating, and activity patterns.[1] It turned out that children of all ages, both boys and girls, identified their parents as the most important role models in their lives. This means *you* have the unique opportunity to make a huge difference in the eating habits and health of your child.

Jean Wiecha, a senior research scientist at the Harvard School of Public Health, says, "Parents can create an environment at the home that encourages good health by having an assortment of healthy foods around, by making sure that there are limits set on television, and having meals as a family in the evening."[2]

Is that challenging? You bet! No doubt on some days you will crave a bag of chips and chocolate for dinner. Or on some mornings you will want to sleep in instead of eating breakfast. But remember: *You* are the person your child most looks to for guidance and direction. What you do, far more than what you say, will influence your child's eating habits.

On the other hand, you don't want to use food as a reward. Promising children dessert if they finish their veggies or giving a child

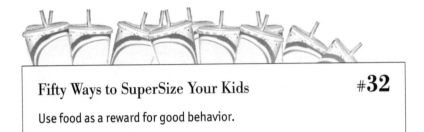

Fifty Ways to SuperSize Your Kids   #**32**

Use food as a reward for good behavior.

a cookie to stop crying sends a mixed message. Using food as a bribe or reward confuses a child's inner signals of hunger and fullness and can cause the child to eat, not when she feels hungry, but when she needs comfort.[3]

Recipe for Success

As your child's parent, you are the person your child most looks to for guidance and direction.

A national survey of parents indicated that while about 70 percent want their children to have good nutrition and eating habits, only 40 percent said they'd succeeded in this area of parenting.[4] Why the discrepancy between desire and success? One reason may be that parents find it difficult to practice these habits themselves. For example, only 51 percent of parents consider it absolutely essential to impress upon their children the importance of exercising and being physically fit. In addition, more than nine out of ten parents say they let their children eat junk food. And 20 percent of parents let their children eat junk food constantly.[5]

Parents often fail to teach good eating habits, and not because they lack information and knowledge. But if we want our children to avoid becoming SuperSized, *we* must model good nutrition and eating habits. Furthermore, it's much easier to teach these principles to

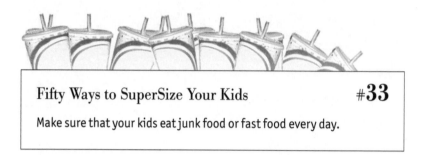

Fifty Ways to SuperSize Your Kids   #**33**

Make sure that your kids eat junk food or fast food every day.

young children as opposed to waiting, as the Larimores did, until their teen years. But even if your kids are older, it's never too late to start down the road to health.

GETTING THE PORTION SIZES RIGHT

We live in a world of all-you-can-eat buffets, super-duper thirst quenchers, and "home of the five-pound burger." Serving sizes are growing bigger each year, along with America's waistline.

So where does a concerned parent start to make a difference? One good place is with appropriate portion sizes. Remember that children aren't small adults, so they don't need adult portions of food.

Food for Thought

"If they have food left on their plate when they say they are done, leave it. It is much better to go into the waste than onto your child's waist."

Lenore Hodges, Ph.D., R.D.
Dietitian at Florida Hospital

It's crazy to plop large quantities of food on a large plate and serve it to a starving child. If you've ever watched hungry children eat, then you know they can pack it down very quickly. And it takes a child's stomach between twenty and twenty-five minutes to let the child's brain know it's filling up.

Also remember that children go through several stages of growth, some that require extra calories and others that seem to require no additional calories at all. And don't forget what we discussed earlier: Children are pretty good at regulating the amount of food they eat, if we don't make a fuss about it.

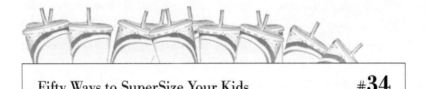

Fifty Ways to SuperSize Your Kids   #**34**

Don't bother to learn the appropriate portion sizes for your child's age.

When working with parents and children struggling with weight issues, Sherri always lets them know that she understands that weighing and measuring food just doesn't work in the real world. So she tries to give them examples of easy-to-eyeball serving sizes they can relate to. Here are a few examples:

- One protein serving is about the size of a computer mouse or deck of cards.
- One tablespoon is about the size of two AA batteries.
- Two tablespoons look about the size of a golf ball.
- One ounce of cheese is equal to four dice.
- One-half cup would fill a cupcake wrapper.
- One cup is the size of a tennis ball.

Of course, the age of your child will determine the portion you should serve. Your two-year-old doesn't need the same serving size as your twelve-year-old! On page 165 is a basic chart to help you figure out the appropriate serving size for your child based on his or her age.

BREAKFAST, THE MOST IMPORTANT
MEAL OF THE DAY

On many early mornings Sherri finds herself at local high schools, talking with students about good eating habits. She always asks, "How many of you had breakfast this morning?" Usually half of the students raise their hands. Then she asks, "What did you have for breakfast?"

This is where it gets interesting.

Among those who had breakfast, about half say they had soda and french fries. Not the best way to start their day!

Many of us think that skipping breakfast is no big deal. We complain that we don't have time, just can't eat early in the morning, or want to save the calories and lose weight. A 2003 survey reported that only 38 percent of study participants ate breakfast every day, although 79 percent said they knew the benefits of eating breakfast.

Recipe for Success

Introduce your kids to the Royal Nutrition Plan. It's simple to remember. Have your child eat breakfast like a king, lunch like a queen, and supper like a pauper!

The American Dietetic Association has reported that up to 40 percent of children aged eight to thirteen skip breakfast. But families dealing with obesity issues have to understand that breakfast is an *essential* part of the game plan. Consider three reasons why breakfast is crucial for your child:

Healthy Portion Sizes

Protein Group

Meat, poultry, f sh, 1 egg, legumes, cheeses, meat analogs, peanut butter, tofu

Age 1-3	**Age 4-6**	**Age 7-10**
2 Servings	2 Servings	2 Servings
(1 oz. each)	(1 1/2z. each)	(2 oz. each)

Substitutes for the protein of 1 oz. of meat: 1 egg, 1 oz. cheese, 1/4up cottage cheese, 1/4up peanuts, ⅛ cup cooked dry peas or beans, 2 T peanut butter.

Dairy Group

Milk (whole, skim, dry, evaporated, buttermilk) and other dairy products

Age 1-3	**Age 4-6**	**Age 7-10**
2 cups	3 cups	3 cups

Substitute for the calcium of 1 cup milk: 1 cup yogurt, 1 ¼ cup cottage cheese, 1 1/2up ice cream, 1 1/4z. (⅛ cup) grated natural cheese, 1 3/4z. processed cheese.

Vegetable and Fruit Group

For vitamin A: Deep yellow-orange or very dark green
For vitamin C: Citrus fruit, melon, strawberries, broccoli, tomatoes, raw cabbage

Age 1-3	**Age 4-6**	**Age 7-10**
5 Servings or more	5 Servings or more	5 Servings or more
(1/4up each)	(1/4up each)	(1/2up each)

Include one vitamin C source daily, and one high vitamin A source at least every other day. Other fruits and vegetables f ll out this food group.

Bread and Cereal Group

Whole grain or enriched bread, cereal, rice, pasta

Age 1-3	**Age 4-6**	**Age 7-10**
3 Servings	4-6 Servings	4-6 Servings

Very active children, teens, adults, and athletes need more for energy. A serving is 1 slice bread, 1 roll, 1/2 cup cooked cereal products, 1 oz. dry cereal.

1. Breakfast revs up children's internal engine, fueling their brains and muscles, so they burn calories more efficiently throughout the day. Eating breakfast means that your child is less likely to be overweight. The University of Massachusetts Medical School found that Americans who routinely skipped breakfast were four and a half times more likely to be overweight.[6] Another study found that children aged four to twelve who frequently ate whole grain cereal had a body mass index close to that recommended for their age group and were at a lower risk for overweight.[7]

Recipe for Success

Eating breakfast helps to control weight by curbing the urge to snack later in the day.[8]

---

2. Children who eat breakfast do better in school. Studies have shown that children who eat breakfast concentrate better, are more creative and alert, and tend to score higher on tests. And according to the American Dietetic Association, children who eat breakfast also do better on tasks involving attention and memory, have fewer visits to the school nurse, and are absent less often.

3. Children who eat meals with their families report better family relationships.

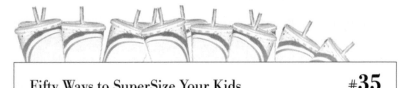

Fifty Ways to SuperSize Your Kids   #**35**

Let your child skip breakfast most days.

Remember that no hard-and-fast rule says you have to eat breakfast food at breakfast. If you prefer eating some of last night's leftovers—as long as they're healthy—go for it! The important thing is to eat something healthy to start off your day.

If your family's breakfast cereal comes loaded with sugar and refined flour, start by choosing a cereal lower in sugar, then make the move to a whole grain, low-sugar cereal (Cheerios, Great Grains, and Wheat Chex are three examples). Think about making oatmeal your new traditional Saturday morning breakfast. Add some nuts and fresh blueberries, and you're good to go!

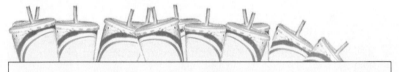

Fifty Ways to SuperSize Your Kids   #36

Buy your kids high-sugar, low-fiber, highly processed cereal and soak it with whole milk.

Here are some other quick, easy-to-fix breakfast ideas:

- Take your favorite whole grain cereal, top with nonfat yogurt and your favorite sliced fruit, and eat it like a sundae.
- Top a whole grain toaster waffle (or whole grain toast) with natural peanut butter and sliced bananas or warm applesauce.
- Try quick-cooking oatmeal topped with fresh fruit and chopped nuts.
- Make a breakfast burrito with a warm corn or whole wheat tortilla, scrambled eggs, low-fat shredded cheese, and salsa. For variety (and more protein), add black or pinto beans.
- Melt a slice of low-fat cheese over a whole grain bagel and have a small glass of 100 percent fruit juice.

- Make your own smoothie using your favorite frozen fruit (without added sugar) and nonfat milk or soy milk. Enjoy with a small handful of nuts for added protein.

LUNCH 101

While many schools have begun to experiment with more healthful lunch foods, your child may still have a hard time eating well at school. Ask for a copy of your child's lunch menu so you will know ahead of time what is available. Consider a few choices you can encourage your child to make:

- Whenever possible, have vegetables or a salad with lunch, even with pizza.
- Drink water, nonfat milk, or 100 percent fruit juice instead of soda or fruit drinks.
- Eat fruit for dessert several times weekly.

If some days have fewer healthful choices, consider having your child take his or her own lunch. Because of the demands on your time, you might be tempted to give your child a prepackaged lunch. While these are convenient and kids love them, they can be high in sodium and fat and low in fiber. Instead, sit down with your child and come up with a list of lunch box favorites. A healthy lunch will include a lean or plant protein, a vegetable, a whole grain, fruit for dessert, beverage, and condiments. Also include appropriate utensils, napkin, and a moistened wipe for cleanup. Here are a few other suggestions to get you started:

- Surprise your child by using a whole grain pita pocket or a whole grain bagel instead of regular bread. These provide more nutrients and fiber.

- If your child loves peanut butter sandwiches, pump up the nutrition by adding thinly sliced strawberries, low-fat granola, or chopped apples.
- Instead of the traditional sandwich, try a wrap. Spread the wrap (a tortilla) with a thin layer of hummus (a garbanzo bean spread that can be purchased at most major grocery stores). Next, add finely chopped vegetables, such as cucumbers, yellow squash, zucchini, and tomatoes. Top with chopped avocado or shredded cheese. Roll tightly or slice into pinwheels and place in an airtight bag.
- Avoid regular processed luncheon meats, which are usually high in sodium and fat. Instead, try sliced turkey breast or lean roast beef slices from the deli.
- Try berries mixed into nonfat vanilla yogurt, topped with chopped nuts, and whole grain crackers on the side.
- Another kid favorite is peanut butter and sliced banana rolled up in a whole wheat tortilla. To keep the banana from turning brown, send a whole banana and a plastic knife so your child can slice it right before eating.
- Instead of a sandwich on white bread, use a whole wheat pita pocket stuffed with your child's favorite chopped veggies. Mix the veggies with low-fat grated cheese and just a touch of salad dressing. To prevent sogginess, put the veggie mix in a separate container and let your child stuff the pita at lunch. Add a handful of nuts and piece of fruit to round out.
- For a simple lunch, pack a hard-boiled egg, whole grain crackers, carrot sticks, and grapes.
- Include a bottle of water, a carton of 100 percent fruit juice, or nonfat milk to complete the lunch.
- You may also need to include additional food as a snack, especially if your child is involved in an after-school program or has an early lunch hour.
- Include a little note, letting your child know that you are thinking of him or her.

Don't forget food safety when packing your child's lunch. Put cold foods in an insulated lunch box and include either freezer gel packs or small frozen juice packs. This is especially important when sending meat or egg sandwiches and dairy products. Keep hot foods hot by placing an insulated bottle in the insulated lunch box. Fill the bottle with boiling water, let it stand for a few minutes, then empty. Place the hot food in the empty bottle. Keep the bottle closed until lunchtime.

It takes a little planning (don't forget to get your child's input!) and it takes a little work (don't forget to let your child help or even do this chore!), but it is well worth the effort to provide your child with a healthful lunch.

WHAT'S FOR DINNER?

Family meals have long been an American tradition. During the past several decades, however, the American family has undergone radical changes—and family meals have changed at the same time.

Yet while most American families have abandoned the traditional "Cleaver family" meal, a whopping 80 percent of American parents still believe it is important.[9] Today's adolescent eats only about one-third of his meals with his family,[10] and up to 32 percent of teens report rarely eating meals with their families.[11]

Why don't parents and children eat together? Two words: schedule conflicts.[12] The American family is busier than ever. In most households both parents work, many times until well past the dinner hour. Children have several extracurricular activities that last into the evening—sports, music lessons, outside classes. And as they get older, they want to spend more time with their friends and develop a sense of autonomy.

Do you find it an increasing challenge to bring your family together for meals? Do you feel tempted to forgo family meals because you can't see how to squeeze one more thing into an already

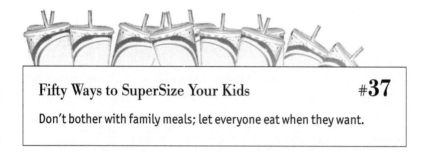

Fifty Ways to SuperSize Your Kids   #**37**

Don't bother with family meals; let everyone eat when they want.

overcrowded day? Before you totally write off family meals, take a look at the benefits of families eating together.

Children from families who eat together have better nutrient intake because they eat more fruits and vegetables and drink more milk. They also eat fewer fried foods and drink less soda.[13] Research has also found that children who eat with their families make better food choices when they don't eat at home and are more likely to eat breakfast.

Other benefits also exist, aside from the nutritional ones. A 2003 survey found that teens who eat five or more meals a week with their families are more likely to earn As in school. They report lower levels of stress. And they are less likely to smoke, drink, or use illegal substances.

As much as possible, keep to a regular schedule for family meals and snacks. *You* may do fine when eating on the go, but this probably doesn't work as well for your children. Remember that a regular routine is not only much better for your health; it's also more satisfying for your child.

Try hard to make mealtimes as pleasant and fun as possible. We all enjoy our meals more and tend to eat better when we face fewer distractions. This is especially true for children. So turn off the TV and mute the ringer on the phone. Surveys have shown that if parents are on the phone or watching TV during meals—even if the kids are right there with them—the children interpret it as not really having a meal with their parents. Why? Because the parents are not focused on talking to them or finding out how their day went. If you're allowing phone calls or other distractions to interrupt your mealtimes, then realize that your children will likely perceive your meal together as *not* really a meal together. So, as much as possible, get rid of distractions. This tells your children that they, and your family meals, are important. We all know that modern life wouldn't be the same without the telephone, but during dinner or after a set time at night, don't answer it. Let the answering machine earn its keep.

When Walt's kids were growing up, he allowed no phone calls during dinner and after a certain time at night. When his kids started moving into upper-elementary and high schools, he and his wife established a phone curfew: No one could make nonemergency calls after 9 P.M. That rule applied to the whole family, Mom and Dad included. The kids had no phones in their bedrooms; they didn't stay up all night talking to a boyfriend or girlfriend; and no one took calls after nine. If the phone rang during dinner or after nine, they let the answering machine get it. Walt and Barb wanted to give their children the message that they were more important than any phone call. Whatever it was could wait.

It will take some planning and forethought to pull off regular, healthful family meals. But it is worth it for the health and well-being of your children.[14] Here are a few tips that might help make dinnertime more enjoyable:

- It is difficult to put a healthy meal on the table if you wait until ten minutes before mealtime to decide what to make. So set aside one hour to plan the menu for the coming week. Then put together your shopping list. This will save both time and money at the grocery store.
- Involve your children in the meal-planning process. Work some of their favorite foods into the menu as often as possible. They will feel that you considered their preferences and will be more likely to enjoy the meals.
- Balance is the key. Have a blend of whole grain carbohydrates, a protein of either animal or plant origin, vegetables, and nonfat dairy products. Serve desserts sparingly.

- Use fruit, nonfat yogurt, or nuts to top off your meal. Consider fruit as "nature's best dessert"! A colorful fruit salad, a baked apple with a dash of cinnamon, or frozen grapes and blueberries can supply just the right amount of sweetness to end any meal.
- When your schedule falls apart, a well-stocked pantry and freezer can be a lifesaver. Have these items on hand: For a quick sandwich, have whole grain bread, lean meats (from the deli counter, not prepackaged), and canned tuna; to a steaming pot of vegetable soup, add whole grain pasta and canned beans and serve with whole grain crackers; for a colorful salad, have washed greens (the darker the better), precut vegetables, raisins, and chopped nuts. Even when you're in a rush, you can put a healthy meal on the table!
- Maximize the appeal of your meals by using herbs and other seasonings (go easy on the salt). And have a mixture of soft and crunchy foods for a variety of textures.
- Try to have two or three courses at a meal; dine instead of merely eating. Getting up between courses to clean off the used plates and prepare for the next course will encourage you to move during the meal, allow you more time to digest your food, and will give the family more time to talk. If you can't do this every evening, then at least do it as many nights as you can. Perhaps you could serve a salad first, then the main course, then some fruit for dessert.
- Stock your kitchen with small plates instead of big plates. Dinner plates have put on a few inches during the past several decades. What used to be a nine-inch dinner plate is now, on average, twelve inches. Try large saucers instead of dinner plates. This will make it easier to control portion sizes.
- Let your children serve themselves. Children tend to serve themselves smaller portions than parents do. In one study, children were offered three sizes of plates, all filled with food. The children tended to eat everything on the plate—but the child who ate off the small plate felt the same degree of fullness as the child who ate off the largest plate.

- Keep an informal diary of what you eat at dinner. (Research shows that the average family eats between nine and ten dinners together per month.) Once you determine the foods that you eat most often, ask yourself, "Which of these do we consider the least healthy? Fried chicken? All-meat lasagna?" Then, as a family, come up with a substitute meal for the next month.

Walt's household replaced all-beef lasagna with a vegetarian lasagna made with soy crumbles and whole wheat pasta—easier and faster to cook. Until then, no one could have gotten a soy crumble past his incisors. But he really could not tell that it wasn't Barb's regular lasagna. Next, fried chicken became a lemon herb chicken that the kids loved. In about six months they changed all their dinners to things they really enjoyed as a family. You have to pick and choose; consider it a longer-term experiment. You really can come up with some outstanding and fun alternatives.

For some easy and practical menu plans, visit our Web site at www.SuperSizedKids.com.

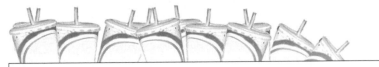

Fifty Ways to SuperSize Your Kids   #**38**

Serve food to your children on large plates and then make them eat every bite.

STRATEGIC SNACKING

Most children need snacks to make sure they get enough calories throughout the day to support growth and to provide essential vitamins and minerals. Snacks are meant to balance out meals, not replace them. Offering healthy snacks at regular times throughout the day (midway between meals) can fill in nutrition gaps. In fact, close to one-fourth of a child's daily caloric intake should come from snacks.

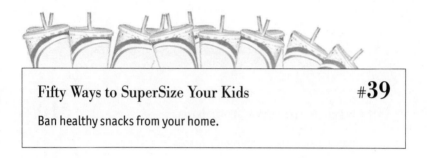

Fifty Ways to SuperSize Your Kids   #39

Ban healthy snacks from your home.

A position paper by the American Dietetic Association, however, reported that most children engage in "mindless" snacking. The result is that they get up to two hundred calories more a day than their counterparts of ten to fifteen years ago.[15] The American Dietetic Association reports that more than 50 percent of children admit to eating while doing something else.

Therefore, you need to eliminate distractions. Turn off the TV, computer, or video game and provide a quiet atmosphere for your child's snack. Snack in the kitchen or dining room. This will help reduce distractions and make it easier for your child not to overeat when snacking.

For a child old enough to prepare his or her own snack, have some healthy fixings within easy reach, in both the pantry and the refrigerator. Store less nutritious items out of sight. Make it easy for your child to snack on healthy foods. Keep fresh, ready-to-eat fruit and nuts on the counter, within easy reach, and place a vegetable sticker on the drawer in the refrigerator where you put the washed and cut vegetables.

We recommend what we call strategic snacking—snacking in a previously determined, well-timed manner that provides children with the energy they need to play and do schoolwork, featuring the nutrients they need to grow and remain healthy. It also helps to prevent overeating, since strategic snacks are "nutrient-dense," not just "calorie-dense." Such snacks must be thought out and planned for. The first thing you grab out of the pantry probably won't qualify as a strategic snack.

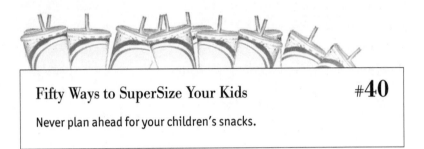

Fifty Ways to SuperSize Your Kids   #**40**

Never plan ahead for your children's snacks.

Strategic snacks combine a "healthy" carbohydrate (fruit, vegetable, or whole grain) with a high-quality protein (lean meat, poultry, fish, nonfat dairy, or plant protein). Why carbohydrates and protein? The carbohydrate provides early energy, while the protein provides energy for later, giving it staying power. Consider these ideas to get you started:

- Whole grain crackers and tuna
- Banana slices and peanut butter
- Raisins and almonds
- Corn tortilla sprinkled with low-fat grated cheese (broil until melted)
- Pineapple chunks rolled up in lean turkey slices
- Apple slices and nonfat yogurt
- Baby carrots dipped in hummus (spread made from garbanzo beans, available at most grocery stores)
- Homemade fruit smoothie (fruit and nonfat milk)

WORKING TOGETHER

Good eating also includes families preparing at least some meals together. When they do so, they enjoy a whole new level of positive interaction. Kids learn all sorts of science, math, and social interaction skills. In addition, kids who help prepare their meals are more likely to eat those meals.

Even incredibly busy families can prepare some meals ahead of time. In a way, it's as if you are preparing your own "fast food." You might say, "We know that we have time on Tuesday to prepare food for our hectic Wednesday and Friday nights. So let's do it!"

A family that prepares and eats meals together can make better decisions about what they're going to eat, when they're going to eat, and how they're going to eat—all of which affect the size of kids. This can also be a wonderful way for your children to develop meal-planning skills so they won't depend on fast food and the pizza delivery-man when they move away from home and have to provide for themselves.

TIPS FOR PICKY EATERS

Worried parents often tell us, "My daughter won't eat broccoli. What should I do?" First, we'd say, calm down; it's probably not as significant a problem as you might think. And then let us offer some information that can help you with your picky eater.

To begin, did you know that even the pickiest eaters tend to grow at normal rates? Children vary in what they want and the amount they eat from day to day. This is all part of the growing process. So don't let the dinner table become a war zone! Remember that your job is to prepare and put healthy food choices on the table. It's your child's job to decide which of the foods he or she will eat and how much.

Consider several tips to keep your picky little eater healthy:

- If your child doesn't like broccoli the first time around, don't worry; keep offering it, and it may become a favorite food. Some children may need to be exposed to new foods as many as fifteen times before they feel ready to try them, and several more times after that before they develop a liking for them.
- Offer meals and snacks only at scheduled times. Sometimes pickiness means nothing more than that your child has snacked all day.
- Serve a variety of foods and include at least one food you know your picky eater enjoys.
- Involve your children with grocery shopping and food preparation. Even young children can wash fruits and vegetables. And it's always more fun to eat something you helped to make.
- Try serving fruits and vegetables more "neutral" in taste. Keep in mind that little taste buds may be sensitive to stronger-flavored foods. At other times use seasonings and flavorings to kick taste up a notch so you don't serve bland food.

As frustrating as your child's picky eating behavior may feel, remember that you, too, dislike certain foods. Most children outgrow their pickiness without any harm to their health. So work with your children. Serve items that you know they enjoy, but continue to introduce them to new, healthy foods.

"HEY, MOM, I'M A VEGETARIAN!"

In the world of today's teens and adolescents it's often considered cool to be a vegetarian. So it's not uncommon for Sherri to get a phone call from the panicked parent of a child who has just come home from school and announced that he or she is now a vegetarian.

The first thing Sherri does is to assure the parent that vegetarian eating is perfectly healthy for their child and can even promote an optimal weight and reduce the risk for many diseases. But she also stresses that vegetarian eating is more than simply avoiding meat and that it's easy to fall into the trap of serving a lot of grilled cheese sandwiches and french fries.

Second, Sherri gives some advice to make sure that the young vegetarian is getting all the proteins and nutrients he or she needs. For a few tips and ideas on vegetarian eating, consult a registered dietitian or go to our Web site at www.SuperSizedKids.com.

Don't be afraid to actively support your child's decision to adopt a vegetarian eating style. Maybe you could learn together, as a family, what vegetarian eating is all about.

SHOULD KIDS GO ON DIETS?

Is it ever appropriate for children to go on diets? Should you ever put your child on Atkins or Sugar Busters or any other similar program? Some school districts have begun to partner with Atkins—and their actions have sparked a big uproar. Why all the fuss?

Because most health experts agree that *diets and children do not go together.*

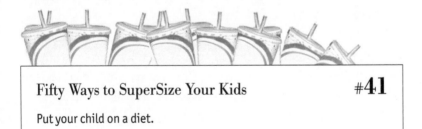

Fifty Ways to SuperSize Your Kids   #41

Put your child on a diet.

As mentioned earlier, Walt actively discourages parents from putting their children on a diet. Data show that dieting in childhood is neither fun nor effective—and may be harmful. Pennsylvania State University researchers, for example, found that young girls who weighed too much and who tried to diet ended up putting on more weight. The unhappier the girls grew with their weight, the more they tried to diet—and the more they failed. Other researchers concur that restrictive dieting is not the best strategy for overweight children. It's much more effective for children to increase their physical activity and change their eating habits. When kids try to diet, more often than not they fail. Most adults who choose to diet do not stay on their diet, either; in fact, they tend to continue with it for an average of just two weeks. So why doom yourself and your children to something very likely to fail? Children who diet are also at a higher risk for eating disorders.

Obesity and the potential for it didn't happen overnight, so we don't have to fix it overnight. Find a long-term strategy that's fun and that will work for you and your family. Again, as you consider the ideas and tips in this book, pick the ones that you think are most likely to succeed, the ones you're most likely to implement—not for only a week or six weeks or six months, but for life.

Remember, children are not little adults. They have unique nutritional needs very different from those of adults. Children who diet set themselves up for big trouble later on.

A REGISTERED DIETITIAN: YOUR NUTRITION EXPERT AND COACH

Does it feel as though the challenges you face might require the help of an expert to get your family on the right eating track? If so, it is important to connect with a nutrition professional truly qualified to help you. Most often this nutrition professional is a registered dietitian.

A registered dietitian has received at least four years of academic training, has had a clinical internship, and has taken a national exam administered by the Commission on Dietetic Registration. Registered dietitians must also maintain their state-of-the-art food and nutrition knowledge by participating in ongoing professional programs. They provide reliable nutritional information, separate fact from fad, and put this information into practical, everyday language.

In many states "nutritionist" and "diet counselor" are not regulated professions. This means that anyone selling diet supplements may refer to him- or herself as a nutritionist without having the education or

qualifications to give sound nutritional advice. When it comes to recommending a nutritional expert to our patients, we recommend a registered dietitian.

Several sources can help you find a registered dietitian: your physician or local hospital, the nutrition department of a local college or
university, or the American Dietetic Association (you can find them
at our Web site, www.SuperSizedKids.com).

FOR BIG RESULTS, START SMALL

How long did it take to build ancient Rome? Who knows—but it took
longer than a day.

Very little that's worthwhile in life can be accomplished overnight.
The same is true with tackling childhood obesity. One important key
to successful family weight management is to *start small* in changing
your nutrition habits—just make sure you start!

All of us are creatures of habit, and good habits take time to kick in
(just as bad habits take time to overcome). Don't try to make wholesale changes in the way you eat; that's a strategy almost certain to fail.
Instead, pick one or two small changes, start with them, and after
you've enjoyed some success, move on and try a few more. Think
"little steps," not "big steps," and you'll be far more likely to reach the
destination of your dreams.

Think of it like this: If you've been walking for ten or twenty or
thirty miles into a swamp, you can't just suddenly decide, "Oh, I don't
like the smell of this swamp," and in that instant find yourself on fra-
grant dry ground. Remember, you're thirty miles in! To get out, you
have to start walking.

If we teach our kids to make small changes now, they can learn
habits that will benefit them for the rest of their lives. Why teach them
to hate dieting when we can teach them to love good eating? Small
steps *work*. But they work only for those who take them.

"It's not about trying to make sweeping overhauls that are
doomed to fail," declares Katherine Tallmadge of the American Dietetic

Association. She says, in fact, that eating just one less tablespoon of fat per day will lead to a ten-pound weight loss in a year.

Uncle Sam agrees. In its Small Step campaign the federal government encourages everyone to give up one soft drink a day, to walk to a co-worker's desk instead of sending an e-mail, to give up a cookie or a candy bar or a bag of potato chips a day, and to take other, similar small steps.

In this chapter we've suggested several dozen simple possibilities that have worked in our families and practices. And we bet you've thought of a dozen more.

So now what?

It's time to sit down and discuss some of these ideas with your spouse and children. Which do they like? Which would they be willing to try? Do you or they have additional ideas about steps you could take that we haven't mentioned? Don't forget: Small changes can result in big health benefits!

Then, once you've finished your family meeting, turn to our eight-week plan in Appendix B, and get started on the small steps that will reap big results for your children.

SIMPLE STEPS THAT WORK

Are you ready to make a few changes today to begin your journey to good eating? Here are a few easy ways to get started:

- Watch portion sizes. Start the meal with small portions. If the child is hungry, going back for seconds is fine, but controlling portion size helps to control calories.
- Resist the urge to go into lecture mode during mealtimes. Make mealtimes fun, not drudgery. Sure, you can make points in your conversation, but don't use family mealtimes to harp on what your children might be doing wrong.
- Slow down! Most adults and children not only eat too much, they eat too fast, even when they have time to relax and enjoy

their food. We can help our children eat more slowly by slowing down ourselves.

- Use small plates. Small plates help you and your child gain control over your portion sizes and trick your minds into thinking you've eaten more than you actually have. (The small-plate strategy will not work, however, if your children consume three or four helpings.)
- Start your meal with a vegetable soup, a fruit dish, or a salad.
- Serve your meal in courses. When everyone has finished the first course, clear the table and wait three to five minutes before serving the second course.
- Encourage your children to taste their food. Having children describe the taste of food slows them down. Most of them do not even think about taste.
- Don't skip breakfast! Better still, get up a little earlier and eat breakfast as a family.
- Educate your child to make the right lunch choices at school. If your child has difficulty finding nutritious food at school, pack a lunch or snacks to go.
- Keep a few items on hand for a fast healthful after-school snack: fruit and veggies ready to eat, peanut butter, low-fat string cheese, nuts, whole grain crackers, raisins, cartons of nonfat yogurt.
- Make sure the healthy snacks in your pantry don't hide on the very top shelf in the back corner.
- Resist the temptation to use food as a bribe or reward. Food should remain a source of nourishment and enjoyment.

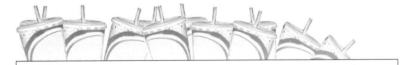

Fifty Ways to SuperSize Your Kids   #42

Train your kids to eat as quickly as possible.

PART THREE

Carry the Torch Beyond the Front Porch

11

BE PART OF THE
SCHOOL SOLUTION

"Dr. Walt," a mom once said during an office visit, "all three of our kids have lost weight, and as they have, I've noticed an improvement in their school performance. Do you think there's a connection?"

"Probably," Walt replied. "My guess is that several things are playing a role, in particular the fact that they feel better and more confident about themselves, combined with positive feedback from their friends."

Research has shown that many factors that contribute to schoolchildren becoming overweight also negatively influence a child's readiness to learn and his or her overall academic achievement. Poor nutrition and lack of physical activity not only help to cause overweight and obesity; they also appear to be connected to significantly lower academic achievement.

THE FRONT DOOR TO
BETTER ACADEMIC PERFORMANCE

Several studies demonstrate that when children's basic nutritional and fitness needs are met, the kids not only perform better in school but also do better on standardized tests. Schools have a critical role in helping students learn and practice good eating habits and in providing the knowledge, motivation, and skills children need for lifelong physical activity.[1] Yet because most of our school districts are getting failing marks in this area, the Institute of Medicine now recommends that they "develop, implement, and evaluate innovative pilot programs for both staffing and teaching about wellness, healthful eating, and physical activity."[2]

Studies in New York have shown that malnutrition too mild to be recognized by parents or most physicians still affected both the intelligence and the academic performance of children. But the studies also noted that this impairment could be corrected through improved nutrition.[3] Another study found that among fourth-grade students those with the lowest amount of protein in their diet had the lowest achievement scores.[4] Moderate undernutrition (nutrient intake that is inadequate or below the optimal levels) can also have lasting effects and may compromise both cognitive development and school performance.[5] Remember the importance of breakfast?

Exercise and physical activity also play a big role in a child's academic performance. Yet 40 percent of U.S. school districts across the country are cutting physical education or recess, believing the extra class time will improve student scores on standardized tests. Many other districts are considering the same. According to Arizona State University researcher Charles Corbin, "Without any question, the No. 1 barrier to physical activity in schools is the perception that time spent in PE and recess will undermine academic learning."[6] It appears this perception may well run counter to the facts.

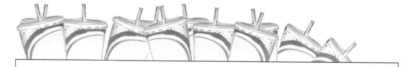

Fifty Ways to SuperSize Your Kids   #43

Support all moves to cut recess and physical education from your child's school.

Studies show that academic achievement improves even when time for academics gets shortened due to physical education activities. For example, a reduction of 240 minutes per week in class time in order to allow children to engage in increased physical activity led to consistently *higher* mathematics scores.[7] Another study correlated SAT-9 test results with a measure called the Fitnessgram and indicated that the physical well-being of students is directly associated with their ability to achieve academically; students with the highest fitness scores also had the highest test scores.[8] Researchers have shown that periods of intense physical activity have positive effects on academic achievement, including increased concentration, improved mathematics, reading, and writing test scores, and reduced disruptive behavior.[9] A growing consensus among researchers, physicians, and policy makers highlights the importance of regular, quality physical education and daily physical activity programs for all students, kindergarten through twelfth grade.

Unfortunately most American school districts have not followed these recommendations. The numbers should trouble us: Only about 25 percent of students attend physical education class daily[10] or partake in any daily physical activity.[11] More than two out of five teens (42 percent) say they would take more physical education classes if available, and only 9 percent would take them less often than they currently do.[12]

Many experts lay the blame at the foot of the country's new focus on standardized tests, including those required by the No Child Left Behind law. School systems, principals, and teachers feel pressured to spend more time drilling kids for tests at the expense of physical activity. But we do so at our kids' and our nation's harm.

Food for Thought

"Everybody agrees that a child's mind is a terrible thing to waste, but we don't seem to mind wasting children's bodies. Maybe we need another law, 'No Child Left on His or Her Fat Behind'!"

Timothy Harper[13]

A HOMEGROWN SUCCESS STORY

Part of the *good* news regarding the nation's childhood obesity crisis is that concerned parents, school leaders, community advocates, and many other individuals and groups across the country have recognized the critical nature of the problem and are taking positive steps to deal with it.

One such example is the Winter Park Health Foundation in the Orlando area, where Nancy R. Ellis served as program director for the Coordinated Youth Initiative. A few years ago the foundation developed an aggressive vision to help its community become the healthiest in the United States by 2007. At that time it adopted children and youth as one of its three primary areas of focus. Since then it has been at work in a growing number of local schools—currently fourteen—to foster and encourage better health.

"We got into this when we started looking into the health connection between nutrition, hydration, physical activity, and their relationship to academic performance," Nancy told us. "That was how we got started doing health promotion activities in our schools."

The foundation's mantra—"Healthy kids make better students, and better students make healthier communities"—provides the guiding light for everything done under the umbrella of the Coordinated Youth Initiative. Programs began slowly, primarily in one pilot school, and evolved over time.

Healthy School Teams

Today every school in the Coordinated Youth Initiative has formed a "healthy school team" comprised of parents, teachers, administrators, and at the high schools, students. As an extra incentive, the high school students who continue to participate on their healthy school team receive free memberships to a local health club.

Once the team comes together, the foundation invests a few thousand dollars in the school. "The biggest thing about the healthy school teams," Nancy said, "is that they're not expensive; we're talking just $6,000 per school."

Of that total, $2,500 is earmarked for a stipend for the team leader (who may be a parent, teacher, or administrator). An additional $2,500 goes for projects with an activity and nutrition focus. The teams also get a hundred dollars a month to spend on various activities of their choice. Each team identifies the areas in health promotion that it thinks afford the best chance for success. So far, every school team has independently decided to focus on nutrition and physical activity. "We allow each school to identify its own priorities," Nancy says, "so then it's theirs, not ours. And that's a critical piece." At monthly meetings with the leaders of healthy school teams, ideas start flying about how to engage students and staff in activities and programs focused on nutrition and physical activity.

"These healthy school team leaders have really caught the vision, and they are absolutely sold," Nancy said. "In fact, this year we had no turnover; they're all coming back next year, even though it requires a lot of extra time. They get a stipend, but they put in a whole lot more time than that."

Ideas, Ideas, Ideas

The healthy school teams have generated scores of creative ideas to help get their schools healthier. Here are some of them:

- The high school held a huge pedometer challenge featuring multiple faculty teams. "We got a chuckle out of it," Nancy said, "because everybody wanted the bandleader on their team; we hear he walks about fourteen miles a day."
- Some schools bought new water coolers or bottles for faculty and students so they could remain hydrated throughout the day.
- One teacher, Jana Ricci, has taught her students to make healthy smoothies. She teaches them to measure ingredients by using their hands as a reference so they can duplicate their work at

home. They use fat-free yogurt, fresh fruit, and 100 percent fruit juices with no additives. One day Jana got a call from a local grocery store manager. He wanted to know what she was doing, because her students were dragging their parents to his store to get the special juices. "Ms. Ricci said I have to have that," they'd say. Eventually the store manager had to expand his fruit juice selections to meet the kids' demands.

- Teachers walk students through making healthy food choices. Kids have to figure out what a serving is and how to measure it with their hands, and what constitutes wholesome fruits, grains, vegetables, and protein. They literally walk through the food pyramid, and at every station they gather up what they should be eating each day from each food group.

- Some schools have organized before-school running clubs that encourage kids to get out and run around the playing field, for which they earn rewards. Other teams have sponsored 5K walks and runs.

- Most schools have "Wellness Wednesday," dedicated to specific activities related to health. They might start with announcements in the morning and offer healthy recipes or ideas for increased activities. At one middle school the team leader, a vice principal, talked the cafeteria manager into eliminating sodas, desserts, and other sugared items from the school cafeteria for a day; then she did a survey of teachers in the period afterward to see if they saw a difference in student behavior. Some schools have a reward system for kids who bring healthy lunches or who buy healthy meals at the school cafeteria.

- One leader of a healthy school team used some of her project money to set up a challenge with the teachers; those who agreed to develop curriculum modules related to nutrition and activity received an extra hundred dollars for classroom supplies.

- The leader of another healthy school team used his project money to purchase Geomats for his PE classes. The mats light up to different patterns—almost like playing hopscotch, except the kids follow lighted patterns. "The kids just love them!" Nancy declared.

- Some schools have sponsored family nights or special student nights at the local YMCA; at one such event about two hundred kids showed up.

- Efforts are progressing on making school vending more health-ful. "The vending income that the high school gets is the only flexible income it has anymore," Nancy explained, "so we're look-ing at ways to create a no-risk clause to see if the principal would be willing to pilot a change in the vending. We're discussing all kinds of ideas that can alleviate his risk. We're working very care-fully to see how we can make it a win for everybody."

- Sue Grafton, president of KidFit America, has worked with the healthy school teams at several schools. They're using their project money to do an exercise fitness program for kids. Sue works with them on daily exercise routines and helps them keep a nutrition log; she also teaches about the importance of ade-quate hydration. "It's a complete program teaching kids how to be healthy," Nancy said. "At one school the kids didn't want to stop when the twelve weeks were up."

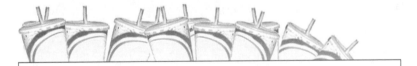

Fifty Ways to SuperSize Your Kids   #44

Encourage your child's school to ignore healthy nutritional and activity habits.

While the teams have developed and implemented far more ideas than these, this will give you a taste for what's happening in the Win-ter Park schools. "They're doing incredibly creative things that are educating the kids and helping to change their behavior patterns,"

Nancy exclaimed. "I can't even keep up with all the things they're doing." And best of all, the teams share their ideas with one another so that an enormous amount of creative cross-fertilization occurs.

The Support of Principals

One key to the success of the initiative, according to Nancy, is that "very quickly we moved to secure the support and cooperation of the principals. We worked really hard to ensure that we were doing what *they* saw as the most critical activities and projects. You have to realize that if you're going to have a program in someone's house, then you need to respect the house rules. If you really want buy-in, then they have to adopt and incorporate the ideas into their own school and community culture."

One strategy that helps to get this buy-in is to show the principals relevant research—article after article and research project after research project that demonstrate a very strong link between nutrition, physical activity, and brain function.

An Environmental Scan

The next big thing on the foundation's docket: a complete environmental scan of the Winter Park schools. The foundation wants to know what currently exists in the way of nutrition and activity options: how long are the lunch hours, how large are the cafeterias, what schools have vending machines (and what types), what kind of playground equipment exists, what sort of physical education classes are offered, etc.

"The biggest thing we're facing with the cafeteria is not just the menu," Nancy explained, "it's lines, it's access, it's the rapidity with which students get their food and the time they have to eat the food."

Since most high school students don't eat breakfast—they're already at school at 7:30 A.M.—Nancy thinks that part of the solution might be to "make some kind of fast breakfast item available on a food cart between first and second or second and third periods." One school, in fact, has already done this.

Some Good Research Data

Over the past two years Nancy has been working with a team of faculty from the College of Health and Public Affairs at the University of Central Florida to develop an integrative research and evaluation model for the schools. "We want to see which of our programs are working," she said. "Do the kids understand what good nutrition is? Are they reporting that their eating habits are changing?"

The foundation is investing a "huge" amount of money in data collection so that it can track what happens to students as they get older. "If we do our job well in the elementary schools," Nancy predicted, "I think we will see that as they get to middle school and high school—and continue to get reinforcement from the healthy school teams—they'll bring their healthier attitudes, values, and behavior with them."

The Real Goal: Culture Change

The ultimate goal of the Winter Park Health Foundation's Coordinated Youth Initiative is to change the school culture so that it leads to a lifetime change in a student's behavior. "The real test will come ten years from now when, I hope, we'll have young people who are healthier and whose health prognosis is much better than when we began," Nancy declared.

It's tough to change a school culture, no doubt about it. But it can be done. Consider just three such examples from the Winter Park experience:

1. All of the healthy school teams want to discourage candy drives to raise money for various groups and organizations. They would much prefer that these drives sell other items or services. But how can you teach a young student to prefer something other than candy? Nancy has one idea. "I can't tell you how touched I was when I drove past one of our schools, probably in midwinter, and read the marquee out front: 'Get Healthy: No Candy at School Week.' That's a culture change, and it's making a very clear statement about where the values at that school are."

2. A parent/school group had scheduled an after-school celebration at a parent's home. The adults had set out sodas for the kids and water for the adults; but the kids drank all the water, leaving the adults with nothing but soda.

3. Another major culture change involved the drive to allow water bottles in the classroom. Just a couple of years ago the practice was banned. But today almost every Winter Park school allows children to take water bottles into the classroom. The change started with convincing staff and faculty that it wouldn't be messy, that the kids wouldn't keep spilling water, that it wouldn't cause excessive noise and activity, and that kids wouldn't keep getting up and down to use the bathroom. The bottom line? *None* of those things occurred. So now, in most schools, kids are carrying water bottles to class and can drink from them whenever they want to.

Next Up: More Family and Community Involvement

The foundation has begun setting its sights on getting families and the community more involved in the schools. "We want to investigate how we can come together as a community to look at the issues of vending and cafeteria," Nancy said, "and how to best influence policy. We're also looking at furthering community engagement; how do we bring businesses into this? Can we get businesses to support some of these healthy school teams?"

So after spending so much energy and money over the past few years, have these various initiatives "worked"? Are the students in the

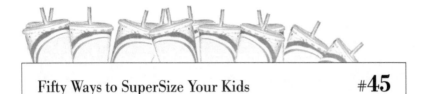

Fifty Ways to SuperSize Your Kids   #**45**

Lobby your child's school to operate plenty of vending machines, stocked with lots of unhealthy foods and drinks.

Winter Park schools getting healthier? Are they dropping dangerous extra pounds?

Nancy believes she'll know more once her developing data collection and analysis programs get online, but already some very encouraging signs have appeared. The schools have reported significant drops in student BMI scores, even as academic achievement scores have climbed. And that's good news not only for the schools involved in the Winter Park Coordinated Youth Initiative but for other schools who are watching.

"The goal is that if you can figure out what works, you share it," Nancy insisted. "That's the bottom line. We're not trying to do something that makes the Winter Park Health Foundation look good; we're trying to do something that will change the community, one kid at a time. And if we can change the prognosis for the most at-risk kids in our community, and thus for all kids, then we've done a wonderful thing. That's really what this is all about."

WHAT PARENTS CAN DO

Winter Park does not have a lock on creative ideas to help our kids get healthier. By working with other interested parents, you, too, can play a vital role in improving nutrition and exercise for the students in your child's school system.

An informed, involved group of parents often leads the way to

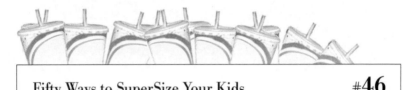

Fifty Ways to SuperSize Your Kids   #46

Refuse to get informed about the nutritional and activity
environment of your child's school.

local improvements, which can not only make healthier families in
your community but also serve as models for state and federal
changes. You probably cannot do all of the following activities, but
you might want to consider a few of them.[14]

1. Visit Your Child's School

Begin by determining what nutrition and physical activity is being
offered to students. Talk to teachers and the principal about your
interest in improving the nutritional value of foods sold and served
in your child's school. Also let staff know about your interest in
improving the physical activity of children. Explain your concerns for
your child's health and the growing childhood obesity epidemic.

Next, determine who makes the food decisions in the school and
contact that person or committee. If you don't find alternatives to
junk food, ask these decision-makers why not. Again, explain your
concern for your child's health and the growing childhood obesity
epidemic. Ask for permission to recruit other parents and students
who share your concern, using a sign-up sheet or a notice in a school
newsletter. Ask if nutrition education is part of the curriculum.

Third, investigate the school policies for physical education and
recess time and ask permission to compare your child's school with
recommendations found in this book or other sources.

Finally, assess your child's school. You'll find a variety of assessment tools on our Web site at www.SuperSizedKids.com. If you do

not have access to the Internet, much of the same information can be found in note 15 for Chapter 11 in the Endnotes section at the back of this book.

2. Brainstorm Options to Begin Correcting What You Find

No one can do everything necessary to bring about needed change, but anyone can start the ball rolling. Take some time to dream up what you might be able to do. For example, you might volunteer to oversee recess at your child's school. Most schools welcome parent involvement. Come up with creative ways to make this a fun, more active part of the school day. Or if you enjoy gardening, you might work with your local school to put in a garden on the school grounds. This is an excellent way to teach children about nutrition and encourage them to try new foods.

3. Build Support and Include Students

After getting answers to your initial questions, assessing your child's school, and looking at what options you have to get the ball rolling, begin soliciting support from other parents and students.

Seek a diverse group of people, including students, who can work together toward a shared goal. With clear goals your group will probably grow as it works on whatever your campaign becomes. You might also look for supporters among teachers, food service staff, a local pediatrician or family physician, a registered dietitian, PTA members, and/or a local businessperson. You can also contact local children's advocacy groups and other nonprofit organizations that might be interested in children's health.

4. Set Early Goals

After forming your group, determine your goals. Learn what other schools have done. If your district does not have a nutrition policy, this may become your goal. We have many examples of school districts with good nutrition policies on our Web site at www.Super-SizedKids.com. Many policies ban soft drinks and junk food altogether. Some policies outline how funds from vending machines will be allocated; some mandate nutrition education in the schools. A policy could require public hearings prior to schools entering into long-term contracts with food and beverage manufacturers. Define your priorities.

5. Meet with Vending Machine Decision-Makers

In some schools, school administrators manage the vending machine program; in others, someone else runs the program. Whoever it is, schedule a time to talk with that person to determine his or her view of the food offered at the school. Whoever runs the vending machine program should be involved in the process. If they fear that a change to healthier options will cause them to lose money, they will resist the change. We have examples of healthful food vending machines at our Web site, www.SuperSizedKids.com.

6. Be Prepared for Objections

"Kids won't eat healthful foods." This is the most common objection, and not just from school officials but from parents as well. More often than not, however, we find that children just haven't been given healthful food choices. Most parents find that once a child tries something, he or she likes it. As long as the food tastes good, most kids will eat it. In San Diego County a school that had been selling candy, chips, and soda wanted to become a "junk-food-free school." Students helped administrators select healthier vending machine

products. The result was vending machines filled with bagels and cream cheese, yogurt, fresh fruit, trail mix, cheese and crackers, and fruit bars. Soda was restricted to 20 percent of the vending slots. During its first year of operation the vending machine brought the school $200,000 *more* in sales and nearly $15,000 in commissions (compared to $9,000 under the old contract). This solution strengthened the budget and also improved the way kids ate.

"Kids won't exercise." Here again, more often than not we find that children just haven't been given healthy and fun activity choices. Most parents and schools find that once a child tries a fun activity, he or she likes it. Most kids have no objection to doing a fun activity. In Toccoa, Georgia, teachers at the Friendship Elementary School began the Fit Kids Club.[16] Guidance counselor Linda Hinson says many of the kids in the school are obese and have high blood pressure. The teachers wanted to help the kids. Soon after the club's formation, twenty-five fifth graders gave up their recess to exercise. Vital signs are taken at the start and end of the program. Each kid in the Fit Kids Club has his or her name posted on a chart. Every day that the kids come, they get a star beside their name. And once they come for ten days, they get a prize; the more they come, the more prizes they get. But for most of the children the real prize is the exercise. The kids come for many different reasons, but they all seem to agree on one reason: It's fun!

"It's too expensive to serve more healthful foods in schools." In the long run the medical expenses of overweight and obese children will far outweigh any expense we might put into providing better food choices for them now. The surgeon general's 2001 report on overweight and obesity put annual obesity-related health care costs at $117 billion nationwide.

"It's too expensive to provide physical education in schools." As with poor nutrition, the long-term medical expenses of overweight and obese children will far outweigh any expense we might incur by providing fun physical activity now. Moreover, not providing physical education may negatively affect our children's school

performance and standardized test scores. Boys, incidentally, are far more negatively affected by not being able to release some physical energy than are girls.

"*We need the revenue from selling soda and junk food.*" Healthful foods can actually earn money. At the North Community High School in Minneapolis, for example, the district worked with a soft drink representative to increase the number of machines stocked with water or 100 percent fruit and vegetable juices. They limited soda to one machine, with limited hours of sale. They also instituted a competitive pricing system, selling water for 75 cents, sports drinks and 100 percent fruit and vegetable juices for $1, and soda and fruit drinks for $1.25. The water machines were strategically placed in high-traffic areas, and students were permitted to drink water in the classroom. What happened? Soda sales went down—but vending profits increased by almost $4,000. The total number of cases of beverages more than doubled from the previous school year, with water becoming the best seller.

Whitefish Middle School in Whitefish, Montana, switched vending machines from soda pop and candy to 100 percent fruit juice, water, and healthy snacks. Before the switch, six to eight kids *a day* received disciplinary referrals immediately after lunch. Since the switch, only one to two referrals occur *a week*. School officials give credit for the change in behavior to the elimination of so much sugar and caffeine in the students' diets. While gross income has declined, net income has not. A postscript: The school recently purchased its own cold vending machine to sell bagels, nonfat milk, and yogurt.

7. Create a Strategy for Success

After building a coalition of supporters, conducting research, and defining your goals, it's time to begin planning a strategy. Talk to community leaders about funding for your ideas. Maybe you, like the folks in Winter Park, can find a local or regional foundation to support your work.

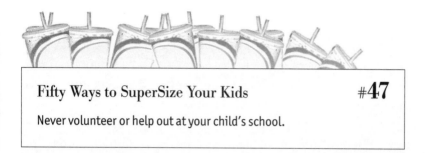

Fifty Ways to SuperSize Your Kids   #47

Never volunteer or help out at your child's school.

Outline a step-by-step process to identify tasks and timelines/deadlines. Then assign each task to a specific individual or subcommittee. Be realistic. Consider the season—it may be difficult to make school contacts or count on parent volunteer efforts during the summer or major holidays. Meet regularly. Communicate between meetings often, perhaps by using a group e-mail list.

8. Scope Out the School Board

Identify your school board members, learn all you can about them, and then enlist them to work toward the common goal of providing a health-promoting nutritional and physical activity school environment for students.

Get to know the local politics of your school board and identify which members are your most likely allies. Attend a few school board meetings for "practice" before making any presentation. Identify anyone you know who might have a relationship with board members—a friend, a neighbor, a business acquaintance.

Start by having a one-on-one meeting with a potential board ally before presenting your idea to the entire board. Ask for strategic advice and help with gaining the support of the remaining board members.

9. Make a School Board Presentation

Try to get better nutrition and physical activities for students on the school board agenda. See if the board has a subcommittee with whom you should meet first. Identify any local leaders who may be able to speak on behalf of child nutrition.

Organize letter-writing and phone campaigns before any formal presentation to the school board so that you can find supporters and make sure they attend the meeting.

Prepare answers to opposing points of view in advance to better address them publicly.

10. Form a Committee

Once the school board passes a nutrition and physical activity environment policy (or anything else you've sought), it's a good idea to create a broad-based committee to oversee how the policy gets implemented.

You'll face many questions and some resistance to change in the beginning, so try to identify a place for people to go to or call if they need clarification on any aspect of the policy. It's probably most helpful to have frequent meetings in the beginning and invite anyone interested to attend.

11. Talk to the Media

Consider media outreach and community relations. The more you can tell people, the more likely you are to gain supporters. Use organization newsletters, flyers, and posters to get out your message. At several stages in the process, newsworthy stories will develop. So nurture relationships with the reporters and assignment editors most likely to cover this issue.

In addition to writing and distributing press releases, write letters to the editor in response to stories that relate to your topic; write an op-ed piece timed to coincide with an important vote at the school board; or request an editorial board meeting to educate your local newspaper on the topic.

Strategic use of media can build support for your effort and give you credibility. Even after a policy gets passed, you can continue to engage the media to help monitor its implementation and share success stories.

12. Watch-Dog the Policy

Once a school food and activity policy gets passed and implemented, it must be maintained. Tight school budgets are the rule these days, and for some, old habits may be hard to kick.

Don't let the school or school board settle for shortcuts. Keep the goal in mind: *an improved nutrition and physical activity environment for schoolkids.* Track and attend important meetings. Develop good relations with food service professionals and physical education professionals. At times you may need to go public again and remind the community of the importance of the new policy, with updates on successes and positive things that have resulted from making children's health a top priority in your schools.

WHAT SCHOOLS CAN DO TO IMPROVE NUTRITION

We join the American Academy of Family Physicians, American Academy of Pediatrics, American Dietetic Association, National Hispanic Medical Association, National Medical Association, and the U.S. Department of Agriculture in calling on schools to recognize the health and educational benefits of healthy eating and the importance of making it a priority in every school.[17] And we agree with the Institute of Medicine's call to school districts to "improve the nutritional quality of foods and beverages served and sold in schools and as part of school-related activities."[18]

It will take groups of parents providing encouragement and leadership to help schools promote good eating for our nation's children. Establishing local policies that create a supportive nutrition environment in schools will provide students with the skills, opportunities, and encouragement they need to adopt these eating patterns. Consider a few basic actions, called for by the organizations listed above, that we think wise:

- Adequate funds can be secured from local, state, and federal sources to ensure that the total school environment supports the development of healthy eating patterns.
- School meals should meet USDA nutrition standards, as well as provide new foods and foods prepared in new ways to meet the taste preferences of students from various backgrounds.
- All students should have lunch periods long enough to enable them to enjoy eating healthy foods with their friends. These lunch periods should be scheduled as near to the middle of the school day as possible.
- Schools should provide enough serving areas to ensure that students don't have to wait too long to get their meals.
- Students, teachers, and community volunteers who practice good eating habits should be encouraged to serve as role models in the school dining areas.
- Foods should come from the five major food groups of the revised Food Guide Pyramid.
- Decisions regarding the sale of foods should be based on nutritional goals, not on profit making.

In addition, schools could aim to meet some or all of the following recommendations:

- All food served or sold on the school property (including food sold by the school, through vending machines, and by outside and student sales) should meet a nutritional standard established by the school system.

- Vending machines accessible to students should not dispense sodas, drinks that contain caffeine or a high concentration of sugar, candy, or similar products. The Los Angeles Unified School District, for example, restricts drinks to "fruit based drinks that are composed of no less than 50 percent fruit juices and have no added sweeteners; drinking water; milk, including, but not limited to, chocolate milk, soy milk, rice milk, and other similar dairy or nondairy milk; and electrolyte replacement beverages and vitamin waters that do not contain more than 42 grams of added sweetener per 20 ounce serving."[19]
- School districts should control all vending machines on their property and should determine the vendors, numbers of machines at each school, their locations, contents, and hours of operation.
- Contracts with vending companies should forbid advertising of food or drink.
- School systems should work to increase the consumption of fresh fruits and vegetables by, for example, establishing salad bars and serving salad shakers (salad and dressing inside a closed plastic container that allows the student to "shake" the salad so it will mix with the dressing) as part of the school lunch program.
- School systems should work to increase the consumption of whole grain foods and snacks.

WHAT SCHOOLS CAN DO
TO IMPROVE PHYSICAL ACTIVITY

Ridgewood High School in New Jersey is trying to "do it right." One parent reported:

My fifteen-year-old son, whose idea of a challenging workout is a new video game, announced after dinner that he was going out for a run. Then my eighteen-year-old daughter, who has always acted as if sweat was her own personal kryptonite, said she would go with him. Since we're a family with tendencies toward laziness, gluttony, and sloth, it was great to see them working out on their own.[20]

How did Ridgewood High School encourage these kids to avoid becoming SuperSized? Coach Chuck Johnson explained that his school is on "the leading edge of a national reform movement loosely known as 'the new PE.'" His classes emphasize collaborative, cooperative activities, such as Project Adventure (a course with a series of daunting physical challenges for teams, such as six students using a rope and a few pieces of wood to work together to ford the creek behind the school), and "lifetime" activities, such as golf, tennis, bowling, aerobics, jogging, self-defense, and rock climbing. Sometimes Johnson gives his classes a Frisbee or a ball and tells them to make up a game. "The only rule is that it has to be aerobic," he said.[21] Educators and parents from schools in Indiana, Vermont, Florida, Maryland, and North Carolina are looking at and adopting some of Ridgewood's innovations.

We join the National Association for Sport and Physical Education in calling for every school to offer at least the following:[22]

- Every student should receive formal instruction in physical education and be involved in physical activity for a minimum of 150 minutes per week in elementary school and 225 minutes per week in middle and high schools.
- Physical education should be taught by a qualified teacher with an earned degree in physical education.
- The physical education class size should be kept to no more than twenty-five to thirty students to ensure safe, effective instruction.
- Adequate equipment should enable every student to participate.
- Indoor and outdoor physical education facilities should be adequate and safe.
- Physical education classes should not be displaced for other activities.

- A written, sequential curriculum should be devised, based on national and/or state standards for physical education.
- An assessment of student learning should be included in the physical education program, complete with meaningful objectives.
- The PE program should provide for maximum participation and successful learning for every student.
- The program should help to systematically develop the physical, cognitive, and social/emotional aspects of the whole student.

BACK TO SCHOOL

The choices we make in our homes have by far the greatest effect on the health and weight of our children. But what happens in their schools can have a profound effect as well. That means that concerned parents must take an interest in what goes on in their children's schools, especially in regard to food availability and exercise options.

Although changes in families and schools provide the foundation for a healthy community, a healthy country also needs your assistance. Some community and governmental changes can provide a great deal of help. And in the last two chapters we'll discuss some ideas that you might want to consider.

12

BRING UNITY TO THE COMMUNITY

When you're sound asleep and floating away in dreamland, what does it usually take to get you awake and moving? A blaring radio? A screeching alarm clock? A sharp jab in the ribs?

How about a wake-up call?

The whole city of Philadelphia received a wake-up call in January of 2000 when *Men's Fitness* magazine named it the fattest city in America. The magazine's editors looked at the city's 30 percent obesity rate, 16 percent exercise rate, surplus of fast-food joints, and lack of fitness facilities and pronounced the metropolis the nation's most bloated.

Fitness-aware Mayor John Street didn't take the news lying down. Shortly after the magazine made its embarrassing announcement, Street announced a citywide shape-up program called 76 Tons of Fun. It challenged Philly residents to collectively lose seventy-six tons in seventy-six days. A Web site encouraged participants to register online, directed them to two hundred "weigh-in sites" throughout the city, permitted them to track their progress, and gave ten simple guidelines for improving their health.[1] It encouraged them to adopt the following healthy-weight habits at a pace of one a week:

1. Find an exercise buddy.
2. Drink plenty of water.
3. Begin to increase your exercise.

4. Eat a variety of fruits and veggies.
5. Eat foods high in fiber.
6. Breathe deeply.
7. Schedule time for rest and play.
8. Eat heavier meals early in the day and lighter meals later.
9. Get plenty of sunlight, which supplies vitamin D.
10. Give someone a reason to smile (good relationships are healthy).

By the end of the challenge in July 2001 the city reported that the more than 25,000 residents who took part had collectively shed about six thousand pounds—not the seventy-six tons the mayor had hoped for, but a great start, nonetheless. To show that it had noticed the contest and to honor the city's efforts, *Men's Fitness* presented the mayor with a Fit City Achievement Award.

"We knew there were things that we could do," Street said, "and that we could create an environment where people were encouraged to exercise and to drink water and to moderate their eating and to exercise a degree of discipline and temperance over what we do. We knew that if we could do that, then we would be a better city and that our citizens would feel better and that we would be a healthier place to live."[2]

The mayor had a lot of help. The School of Culinary Arts at the Art Institute of Philadelphia, for example, helped more than a dozen of the city's restaurants provide healthier menu selections. Several other organizations, including the NBA's Philadelphia 76ers, Time Warner Cable, and Subway, sponsored the program.

Philadelphia police officer Juan Delgado heard the mayor's call and decided to join the challenge. Why? "One day I was patrolling in my vehicle with my tie on and the collar buttoned," Delgado said, "and it was so tight around my neck I felt like I was choking—and it was a 19.5-inch collar, so I couldn't go any bigger. It made me really frustrated, and I just said, 'Okay, that's it. It's time to lose this weight.'" At the beginning of the challenge the five-foot-six Delgado weighed 212 pounds; by the end he had dropped to 148 pounds.[3]

Oh, and one more thing: In its next "fattest city" edition *Men's Fitness* excused Philadelphia from the top spot while a red-faced Houston took over that honor.

IT TAKES A COMMUNITY

Many experts believe that challenges and programs like the one pioneered in Philadelphia are crucial for getting our communities and children back in shape. And, fortunately, such programs are popping up all over the country.

Delia Rochon, director of Utah's Intermountain Health Care Healthy Community initiative, believes that the key to creating any successful program depends on members of the community leading and owning that program. "People tend to listen to someone who they agree with," she said. "We respond better with people who are like us, who live in our community and understand our values and concerns."

And when those people work together for the common good, there's no telling what might happen. "A basic premise of the Healthy Community movement is that well-informed people, working together in an effective process, can make a profound difference in the health and quality of people's lives within the communities," Rochon declared.[4]

Food for Thought

"A basic premise of the Healthy Community movement is that well-informed people, working together in an effective process, can make a profound difference in the health and quality of people's lives within the communities."

Delia Rochon
Director, Utah's Intermountain Health Care Healthy Community

Not to give Philadelphia a big head, but various groups in the city really appear to be "getting it." Alarmed by sobering statistics regarding childhood obesity, spurred by concern about a potential couch potato generation, and motivated by the mayor's 76 Tons of Fun, community health clubs, gyms, and Ys there (and in other places) began to focus on children, tweens, and teens. As a result, kids began dancing, spinning, sweating, walking, and kickboxing.

Town Sports, one of the nation's largest health chains, operates the Philadelphia Sports Clubs and its sister gyms in New York, Boston, and Washington, D.C. One of its newest programs, a youth sports conditioning program designed for tweens, will feature a circuit training workout.

"We are really trying to get that age group," said Kate Hennigan, director of Town Sports International's Sports Clubs for Kids. "We see the void. We see the need."[5] Others in the region are aiming at improved activity and nutrition for kids. The Camden County YMCA, for example, started "ramping"—the hot new thing in fitness. Participants in ramping use an inclined board to build leg strength. One class will be designed specifically for tweens. And the Y has applied for grants to develop a program for overweight youths.

The Northeast Family YMCA in Philadelphia is starting Healthy Kid Zone, a fitness and nutrition program for six- to eleven-year-olds, in conjunction with the Holy Redeemer Health System. About two years ago it started Kid Fit, an exercise program for eight- to twelve-year-olds. And an athletic club is using Instyle Fitness—a revamped and way cooler version of its earlier Girls Club—to attract tweens and teens.

The Deltona YMCA in Orlando plans to start offering Get Real Weight Management, a family-oriented program that focuses less on losing weight than on learning health-promoting new behaviors. "We want to educate families on all the factors that play a part in a person's weight: activity, nutrition, even social and emotional factors," said Patti Stephens, wellness coordinator. "Our goal is to help them incorporate healthy new behaviors into their lifestyles. And we want to help them understand that losing weight has to be a family affair, especially if children are involved."

Communities aren't just ramping up programs aimed at getting our kids active in the gym. Many students are participating in an American Cancer Society program called Generation Fit. Through Generation Fit, students aged eleven to eighteen take part in community service projects that promote more physical activity and better eating habits among their friends and families and in their schools and communities. The young activists themselves come away better educated about good nutrition and the need to stay physically active. At one U.S. middle school a group of students worked to have their favorite healthy foods added to the cafeteria menu.

Coaches, counselors, and youth group leaders can easily run a Generation Fit program. The sponsoring group gives several ideas and suggestions, clustered in five areas:

- Food for Thought: Trying New Recipes in Your Cafeteria
- Message Magic: Selling Healthy Eating and Physical Activity
- Lending a Helping Hand: Planning Meals for Those in Need
- Team Up for Good Health: Improving Habits with a Partner
- Let's Get Moving: Making Physical Activity a Priority in Our Community

Students tailor these ideas to the needs of their own schools and towns. One group prepared a meal for a homeless shelter. Another group of sixth graders taught good health habits to younger students by taking them on walks and giving them healthy snacks. Children who participate in Generation Fit also learn how to plan a community action, work together in a group, and carry out their plans, all with the help of adult leaders.[6]

It's all part of a national trend and, from some quarters, a wake-up call followed by a summons to action. In fact, the American Cancer Society (ACS) has issued a national call for communities to remove any barriers or policies that prevent people from enjoying a healthy lifestyle.[7] The ACS understands that kids who are more active and who eat better not only will dramatically reduce their chances of becoming SuperSized but are also much less likely to develop cancer.

We agree with the ACS Recommendations for Community Action, which state, "Communities should work together to create a healthy environment where everyone has access to healthy food choices and safe places to be active." The ACS recommends that communities increase access to healthful foods, not just in schools but at the work site and also in the community. It also recommends that communities provide safe, enjoyable, and accessible environments for physical activity in schools and for transportation and recreation in communities.

The prestigious Institute of Medicine released a report in late 2004 in which it encouraged the establishment or revision of zoning ordinances and comprehensive plans to include or enhance sidewalks, bike paths, parks and playgrounds, and other recreational facilities.[8] Communities can play a huge role in this battle!

WHAT COMMUNITIES CAN DO

Did you walk or bike to school when you were a child? Thirty years ago more than 66 percent of all children walked to school.[9] Walking or biking to school gives children a sense of freedom and responsibility, allows them to enjoy the fresh air, and provides opportunities to get to know their neighborhood while arriving at school alert, refreshed, and ready to start their day.

Yet today most American children are denied this experience. In fact, only 13 percent of American children walk or bike to school.

Marin County, a picturesque community north of San Francisco, boasts many historic small towns and miles of open space. Despite Marin County's low population growth, traffic had grown increasingly worse, with 21 percent of the morning commute accounted for by parents driving their children to school. As a result, traffic congestion had increased around schools, which prompted even more parents to find it safer to drive their children to school, rather than allowing the kids to walk. In fact, surveys indicated that 73 percent of students commuted to school by car, 14 percent walked, 7 percent biked, and 3 percent arrived by bus.

In August 2000, local leaders, armed with funding from the National Highway Traffic Safety Administration, began to develop a national model program called Safe Routes to School. The popular program, designed to promote walking and biking to school through education and incentives that show how much fun it can be, is quickly spreading across the United States and Canada. The program also addresses the safety concerns of parents by encouraging greater enforcement of traffic laws, educating the public, and exploring ways to create safer streets.

To demonstrate the benefits of Safe Routes to School, parents and community leaders in Marin County recruited nine pilot schools in four locations. Each school received guidance, forms, newsletters, and other promotional materials.

In two jurisdictions schools got together to form citywide task forces to study engineering solutions aimed at increasing safety on routes to schools. They hired a transportation engineer to assist in developing these plans. Every school held periodic Walk and Bike to School Days and participated in the Frequent Rider Miles contest, which rewarded children who came to school walking, biking, by car pool, or by bus.

By the end of the pilot program, organizers noted a 57 percent increase in the number of children walking and biking to school and a 29 percent decrease in the number of children arriving by car (those not in a car pool).[10]

The community of Plano, Texas, had a more tragic wake-up call that motivated it to seek change. In 1998 eleven-year-old Matthew Brown rode his bicycle across a quiet street in front of a truck that had come to a complete stop behind a stop sign. Matthew, believing the truck had spotted him, rode from the sidewalk into the street. The driver never saw Matthew and struck him, killing him instantly.

Matthew's tragic story gripped his community and provoked par-

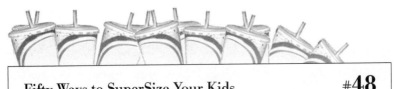

Fifty Ways to SuperSize Your Kids   #48

Even if it's geographically possible, don't walk your children to school or let them walk to school.

ents, physicians, a hospital, and teachers to band together to promote a comprehensive bicycle safety program for Plano. The story also captivated the entire state of Texas, and before long a legislative package to ensure the safety of children walking or biking on Texas roads surfaced. To honor Matthew, legislators gave his name to the bill.

In June 2001 Texas governor Rick Perry signed the Matthew Brown Act into law. Gayle Cummins, executive director of the Texas Bicycle Coalition, quickly pointed out that the success of the legislation depended on a unique coalition of cyclists, parents and teachers, and the medical profession. "The fact that everyone came together and worked so hard to make the Matthew Brown Act a reality is a testament to the genuine concern these groups have for children's safety," she said. "Everyone agrees that bicycling is an important part of children's lives and that it is up to us to make sure they can use bikes to get around safely."[11] Thus a small number of parents in Plano not only increased the safety of physically active children in their community but encouraged the same thing throughout their state.

Food for Thought

"Everyone agrees that bicycling is an important part of children's lives and that it is up to us to make sure they can use bikes to get around safely."

Gayle Cummins
Executive Director, Texas Bicycle Coalition

And it's not just suburban communities that have become concerned about the safety of kids who want to bike to school or become more physically active in other ways. From 1996 to 2000 New York City introduced a Safe Routes to School program in the Bronx. The project showed the city how to do the community education, planning, and consensus building needed to generate strong support for traffic calming around schools and increase the number of kids walking to school.[12] The project generated strong public interest and support from the Bronx delegation to the city council. It took parents and city officials six years to get the program off the ground—but it's making a difference.

These successes—which combined the energies of parents, community leaders, and public policy experts—have brought positive changes in many communities. And as we've emphasized again and again, this type of help couldn't come at a better time in our country's history.

Could you be a catalyst in your area for similar initiatives?

WHAT YOU CAN DO

With more than 130 million Americans working, many parents spend the majority of their days in the office. Since kids follow where adults lead, employers can join these efforts to improve community health by offering healthful food options in vending machines and cafeterias, inexpensive access to a gym, and work-based health programs like the American Cancer Society's Active for Life Program. Parents who learn healthful habits at work are likely to model them for the kids at home.

Healthy parents can influence not only their own kids but kids in the community. Starting in 1997 with just two small groups of parents representing two U.S. schools—and growing to involve more than three thousand schools in 2004—the Walk to School Day is bringing together community coalitions across the country to push

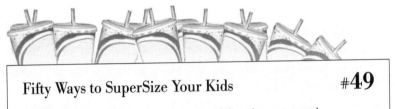

Fifty Ways to SuperSize Your Kids   #49

Neglect good nutrition and physical activity where you work.

for safety improvements for children who walk and to increase physical activity among children.

In 2003 Walk to School Day achieved several victories, ranging
from the announcement of a multimillion-dollar grant to improve
street safety around schools, to the addition of sidewalks as a result of
successful parental rallying. Even communities in which the majority
of students cannot walk to school used the day to kick off year-round
walking-at-recess programs.

"That's great," you may be saying, "but what difference can *I*
make?" Don't sell yourself short! Just one person can make a difference by helping to implement the following ideas:

- Start a walking club at lunch, before work, or after work.
- Obtain information from the Safe Routes to School Program.
  You can find more information on our Web site at www.Super-
  SizedKids.com.
- Organize a Walk to School Day. We have information on our
  Web site about how to do this.
- Examine your neighborhood and determine how friendly your
  streets are for walkers. Here's part of one list recommended by
  the National Safety Council (you can find more detailed check-
  lists on our Web site):
  - Did you have room to walk?
  - Was it easy to cross streets?
  - Did drivers behave well?
  - Was it easy to follow safety rules?

- Could you and your child cross at crosswalks or where you could see and be seen by drivers? Stop and look left, right and then left again before crossing streets? Walk on sidewalks or on shoulders (facing traffic) where there were no sidewalks? Cross with the light?
  - Was your walk pleasant?
- Organize a team for local runs, fund-raising walks, or a corporate challenge event.
- Find speakers for noontime seminars on nutrition, fitness, or weight loss.
- Add healthful snacks to the menu for company events. Try baked chips or baked pretzels instead of regular chips, a fresh fruit or veggie tray, and frozen yogurt with fruit toppings instead of ice cream sundaes for a celebration.
- If you work for a medium to large company, check with the human resources department to see if there are discounts available on gym, YMCA/YWCA, or health club memberships. Also see if there are fitness or nutrition seminars available.

Perhaps you've also noticed that rapid urban and suburban growth has tended to reduce the number of parks and recreation facilities available, thus taking away prime places to exercise. Voice your concerns by voting to preserve parks and green space. Here are a few ways you can help to make change happen more quickly:

- Start a community watch group to improve safety for walkers and bikers and especially children.
- Encourage local planning boards to install more sidewalks, crosswalks, and traffic lights to make walking safe in your neighborhood. You can attend meetings or talk to board members about your concerns.
- Support restaurants in your area that have healthful food options and offer nutrition information, especially calorie counts. In early 2004 a St. Petersburg, Florida, restaurant chose to redesign its

children's menu. It expanded its selections to include grilled salmon and chicken, steamed vegetables, and fruit for dessert. Much to the surprise of the restaurant, these new offerings became a big hit. And because 40 percent of the children who eat here order these more nutritious items, they will stay on the menu.

■ Support local farmers' markets.

At our Web site, www.SuperSizedKids.com, we have plenty of free guidance and informative materials to help you and your friends brainstorm about how you could create a healthier community where you live.

IF PHILADELPHIA CAN DO IT . . .

Nobody wants to end up number one on the *Men's Fitness* annual list of the fattest American cities. Philadelphia didn't care for that kind of exposure, and neither did Houston.

Philadelphia took action by organizing its 76 Tons of Fun campaign. And what did Houston do? It sent representatives to the City of Brotherly Love to take notes on its slim-down project.

"It helped give our people some really good ideas," said Corey Ray, who worked with Houston mayor Lee Brown. "We hope to have a similar plan in the near future."[13]

Any community can do the same—even yours. And who knows? You might be just the person to help get it started.

13

BATTLE OF THE BULGE ON THE STATEHOUSE STEPS

Louisiana, Mississippi, and West Virginia. Do you know what all three have in common? Hint: It's nothing to brag about.

According to Dr. Julie Gerberding, director of the Centers for Disease Control and Prevention, these three states are the fattest in the country, with fully 25 percent of their residents qualifying as obese. "It is a catastrophe in our country," she said. "Unfortunately, poor diet and a lack of exercise have almost caught up with tobacco as being the leading cause of death in the United States."[1]

Gerberding's comments in late 2003 spurred many lawmakers nationwide to propose legislation that, they hoped, would begin to stem the tide of the national obesity epidemic.[2]

Louisiana began an experiment in which the state agreed to pay for a few government employees' gastric bypass surgery (stomach stapling) to see if the procedure reduced health care costs. Schools were required to have physical education programs (prior to this, Illinois was the only state in the Union with laws mandating such classes). Mississippi encouraged, but did not require, physical education classes in its schools.

West Virginia saw billboards sprout up across the state, featuring photos of bulging stomachs accompanied by messages exhorting readers to "Put Down Chips & Trim Those Hips." No wonder: Medical costs for state employees had more than doubled since 1995, rising from $37 million to $78 million—nearly a fifth of the employees'

$400-million health plan. And the state agency that insures public employees started offering exercise benefits and diet counseling. "If we don't get a handle on this, this generation of kids coming up will have a shorter life span than their parents," said Nidia Henderson, wellness manager at West Virginia's Employees Insurance Agency. "That's scandalous!"

Food for Thought

"If we don't get a handle on this, this generation of kids coming up will have a shorter life span than their parents. That's scandalous!"
Nidia Henderson
Wellness Manager,
West Virginia's Employees Insurance Agency

You may not live in one of the "fattest states," but chances are something good is happening where you live, too. Arkansas, for example, named six schools in which children would be tested for their BMI, with the results sent home. Some experts say that regular tests like this should be mandatory nationwide. We believe a child's BMI and blood pressure should be recorded on every child's report card every quarter or semester.

In this final chapter we will survey some recent legislative efforts, as well as a few scientific advances, aimed at combating obesity. And we'll also make a few recommendations of our own.

IT'S TIME TO SHUT DOWN ADVERTISING OF UNHEALTHY FOODS TO KIDS

They're charming, cute, cuddly, adorable, and appealing. And they're trying to hook your kids—even babies—on junk food, for the rest of their lives.

"They" are any of a wide range of youth icons, from Toucan Sam to characters on public television, thought up by marketers in an effort to win kids' attention and their parents' money.

This is the message delivered around the country by psychologist and author Susan Linn, who has written extensively about the effects of commercial marketing on kids. "I know a woman—a very educated woman—whose child's first words were 'Elmo, Nemo, and Coke,'" she says. "Preschoolers can't tell the difference between a commercial and a television program. And until the age of eight, they can't understand persuasive intent. They can't understand the concept of selling. They don't get it. They can't defend against it. And it's not fair we're doing this to them."[3]

A 2002 World Health Organization report concluded that the heavy marketing of "fast food and energy-dense, micronutrient-poor foods and beverages" is a "probable" causal factor in weight gain and obesity.[4] The following year the most comprehensive study of its type conducted to date found that advertising *does* affect food choices and *does* influence dietary habits.[5]

Linn says marketers target even infants in hopes they'll identify with a certain brand and remain loyal to it as they grow older. She cites a wide range of products, including what she described as junk food, marketed by cartoon characters such as Dora the Explorer and Blues Clues. She reports that books for babies have been designed to look like M&M's packages. She says these promotions are intended to make babies associate the candy with the comfort of their parents' voices as they read to them.

"It's a way of getting into babies' brains," said Linn. "That's what we're up against. A lot of Americans believe parents can just say no. But I believe parents need help. We need to address it as a society."

We agree. And so does the nonprofit Center for Science in the Public Interest (CSPI). In a recent report, it concluded, "Food marketing aimed at kids undermines parental authority and helps fuel the epidemic of childhood obesity."[6] According to CSPI, "The volume and variety of marketing techniques has exploded as food marketers seek new ways of bypassing parents and directly influencing kids' food choices. Regrettably, most of the foods marketed directly to children are high in calories and low in nutrition."

Margo Wootan, the director of nutrition policy at CSPI, says, "SpongeBob Squarepants, Winnie the Pooh, Elmo, and even sports stars like Jason Giambi are enlisted to push low-nutrition foods on kids."[7]

Food for Thought

"Doctors call the explosion in [childhood] obesity an epidemic, but food corporations call it a business plan. Kids are not stupid. They know the adults are preaching health while selling a generation out to America's junk-food culture."

New York Daily News
November 30, 2004

Consider just a few examples highlighted in the CSPI report:[8]

- Krispy Kreme's Good Grades program offers elementary school kids one donut for each A on their report cards. CSPI points out that some states wisely prohibit or discourage using food as a reward for good behavior or academic performance.
- The Oreo Adventure game on Kraft Foods' Nabiscoworld.com Web site is one of many corporate "advergames." In this video game children's "health" is reset to "100 percent" when they acquire golden cookie jars on a journey to a Temple of the Golden Oreo. The Oreo Matchin' Middles shape-matching game, produced with Fisher-Price, turns playtime into a chance for companies to cultivate brand loyalty and sell junk food.
- Pepsi's Web site profile of New York Yankees baseball star Jason Giambi prominently displays his quote that "I usually have several Pepsis each day—it really lifts me up." Thus a junk-food marketer links consumption of its product with fitness.

- Cap'n Crunch Smashed Berries cereal—which, predictably, has no berries at all—encourages overeating in its magazine advertisements. Once such ad in *Nickelodeon* magazine reads, "Kids smashed 'em in the factory so you can fit more in your mouth."

In the 1970s and 1980s the Federal Trade Commission considered restrictions on junk-food advertising aimed at kids, but those efforts got blocked by the food, toy, broadcasting, and advertising industries. We believe now is the time to set standards on what foods may be marketed to kids through the media and in schools.

IT'S TIME TO STRENGTHEN FOOD LABELING

The Nutrition Labeling and Education Act, signed into law by President George H. W. Bush in 1990, requires comprehensive, consistent food labeling on almost all packaged foods sold at supermarkets, convenience stores, and other retail stores. Three-quarters of adults report reading and using food labels,[9] and using food labels is associated with eating more healthful foods.[10] About half (48 percent) of these people report that the nutrition information on food labels has caused them to change their minds about buying a food product—a 50 percent increase over the number in a survey conducted before the new food labeling law went into effect.[11]

We believe that strengthening food labeling is likely to yield significant health and economic benefits. And we're not alone. The FDA estimated that just the simple requirement of listing trans fat on packaged-food labels would save 2,100 to 5,600 lives a year and $3 billion to $8 billion a year in health care costs.[12] The USDA has also estimated that the economic benefits of extending nutrition labeling to fresh meat and poultry would save $62 million to $125 million per year.[13] These and other facts led the Institute of Medicine to recommend that the food, beverage, and entertainment industries should voluntarily develop and implement guidelines for advertising and marketing directed at children and youth. It also recommends that Congress give the Federal Trade Commission the authority to monitor compliance with the guidelines and establish external review boards to prohibit ads that fail to comply.[14]

GREAT BRITAIN IS BEATING US TO THE PUNCH

Regulators in Great Britain have announced plans to work with food manufacturers and supermarkets to introduce, by early 2006, a clear coding system for foods so that consumers can understand at a glance what is healthy and what should be eaten only in moderation. They plan to "develop a simple code for processed food to indicate fat, sugar and salt content for shoppers."[15]

The British government proposes voluntary action by industry to reduce levels of sugar and fat in processed foods and to end bigger portion sizes. Already, "overwhelming support for some restrictions on the marketing of unhealthy food and drinks to children" exists in Great Britain. We suspect the same is true in the United States.

And what if volunteer actions don't work? The Brits say, "Legislation may follow if there is no change in the nature and balance of food promotion by early 2007."[16]

What approach might they try? It's called the Traffic Light System. Red, orange, and green symbols would be used to help shoppers quickly determine how healthy their products are.[17] In a report that criticized the government, food manufacturers, and advertisers for failing to do enough to fight obesity, a House of Commons Health Committee recommended the food industry be given three years to voluntarily implement measures, including the informational symbols. If companies fail to do so voluntarily, the government should require them to, the lawmakers said.

Under the Traffic Light labeling system, foods dense in calories, saturated fat, simple sugars, or salt would have to post a red light on their labels; healthier options would get a green light. One supermarket chain in England has announced it would try the system. It said it would use the labels to warn shoppers of unhealthy foods. "We've listened to our customers, and they find current labeling confusing," says Tesco director Tim Mason. "We think the eye-catching traffic light system may be an easy, open and honest way of labeling our products so customers can see exactly what they're eating."[18]

We think it's time for such a system in the United States, despite the outpouring of resistance to be expected from advertisers and those who sell them space in a wide variety of media.

IT'S TIME TO STRENGTHEN FOOD LABELING IN FAST-FOOD RESTAURANTS

Unfortunately the Nutrition Labeling and Education Act of 1990 explicitly exempted restaurants. Under current law, restaurants must make nutrition information available only when they make a health or nutrient-content claim for a food or meal. If a menu board claims that a sandwich is low-fat, for example, the restaurant is required to have available, somewhere in the store, information about the fat content of that sandwich. Unlike for processed foods, whose nutrition information must be determined by laboratory analysis, nutrition information regarding restaurant claims may be determined from nutrient databases, cookbooks, or "other reasonable basis."

Some restaurants, particularly fast-food chains, provide brochures or posters with nutrition information regarding their menu items. Several fast-food chains, however, provided in-store nutrition information only after state attorneys general and consumer groups applied some pressure. In 1986 state attorneys general from several states, including Texas, New York, and California, negotiated an agreement with McDonald's, Burger King, Jack in the Box, KFC, and Wendy's, to provide nutrition and ingredient information in their restaurants.

We see a number of problems with the current voluntary system for providing nutrition information in chain restaurants. In fact,

---

Food for Thought

"The nation's ongoing, literally sickening slide into mass obesity can be halted, but not unless we stand up to the food industry."
New York Daily News
November 30, 2004

---

most chain restaurants do not provide such information. McDonald's and Burger King, to their credit, are the exceptions. A 1997 survey of the largest chain restaurants found that two-thirds (65 percent) do not provide customers with any nutrition information (including on menus, menu boards, pamphlets, table tents, or posters).[19] And often those that do provide the information do so in large, complicated tables listing everything from protein and cholesterol to iron and vitamin A. These tables can be hard to use because they present an overwhelming amount of information in small print for every food item. And not many busy customers want to lose their place in line to try to interpret a poster chock-full of small print.

Worst of all, as time and experience have proved, it is unlikely that a voluntary system will prompt many more restaurants to provide nutrition information. Two-thirds of the largest chain restaurants believe they do not have a responsibility to provide nutrition labeling.[20]

This is unfortunate, for one older study, done in a cafeteria setting, showed that posting signs indicating the calorie content of available foods significantly decreased the number of calories purchased.[21] An unpublished evaluation of a menu labeling program at four northwestern table-service restaurants also found that calorie labeling on menus led to entrée selections lower in calories.[22]

We believe Congress and state or local legislatures should require food-service chains with ten or more units to list the calorie, saturated and trans fat (combined), and sodium contents of standard menu items. Where space is limited, restaurants that use menu boards should be required to provide at least calorie information next to each item on their boards.

We also believe that labeling should be required for foods and beverages sold "to go" at food retailers such as cookie counters in shopping malls, vending machines, drive-through windows, and convenience stores. Further, nutrition information should be required to be listed as prominently as price and other key menu information. The Institute of Medicine joins us in urging restaurants to provide calorie content and other nutrition information.[23]

IT'S TIME TO JUNK JUNK FOOD AT SCHOOLS

As we were writing this book, state legislatures across the United States were considering measures that would wage an attack on junk food in vending machines at their public schools. There are at least twenty-eight states considering such legislation, and at least five other states have imposed restrictions on the snacks students can buy, according to the National Council of State Legislatures.

Why? It's simple. More than three quarters of the snacks and drinks sold in school vending machines have poor to no nutritional value—and most are actually unhealthy.

These states are examining ways to encourage healthy vending machine choices at school. One of the more popular options is to empty those machines of sugary soft drinks and high-calorie snacks and replace them with healthy choices. As we've discussed earlier, surveys show healthy snacks generate just as much money for schools.

Nevertheless, many times local school boards are uncomfortable making this type of change and we feel it is reasonable for state legislators, with the support of those who love and care for kids, to step up to bat and require vendors to put nothing but healthy snacks in machines at public schools.

To see a lengthy list of likely objections to our proposal, check our Web site at www.SuperSizedkids.com. But here we'd like to dispense with just two:

"It is not the job of the state legislatures or school boards to determine what kids eat; that is the role of parents." While this responsibility does

belong primarily to parents, it becomes everyone's responsibility when children eat meals away from home. States and schools must create the best possible learning environment for students. Healthy children grow into a productive workforce, with dietary habits that can last a lifetime. Good nutrition helps a student's academic achievement. A study by the Tufts University Center on Hunger, Poverty and Nutrition Policy reported a link between inadequate nutrition during childhood and cognitive development and productivity in adulthood. Findings also examined the impact that undernourishment has on the children's behavior, their school performance, and their ability to concentrate and complete tasks. Similarly, when children eat a well-balanced meal, such as a school breakfast, they have higher sustained energy levels than children who select foods from only one or two food groups, which are often high in sugar or fat.[24]

"We do not believe in state mandates to local schools." "Local control" in education is a powerful argument for many people. Legislators may say that they oppose issuing state mandates to local schools. This is a health issue, however, much like the asbestos threat that surfaced in schools several years ago. All children need to be protected from the health threat of unlimited availability of high-fat, high-sugar food in their schools. Many states invest significant resources in administering the federal breakfast and lunch programs, creating good nutrition environments, and implementing nutrition curricula. This investment is jeopardized by the increased availability of junk food in schools. The state also picks up much of the tab for the millions annually spent on treating obesity-related illnesses. And that's something we must tackle immediately.

IT'S TIME TO CONSIDER A WIDE VARIETY OF OTHER PROPOSALS

Many national groups have made recommendations for consideration at a local, state, or national level. One that we heartily recommend is changing state transportation policies to encourage physical activity among adults and children. If your state is one of the thirty that have constitutional or statutory restrictions on using state gasoline taxes on anything other than highways,[25] you could work to change the law to allow gas tax funds to be used for bike lanes, walking trails, wider sidewalks, and other infrastructure that supports physical activity. On our Web site we have an example of a relevant constitutional amendment from Maine.[26]

We also believe that the cost of health and life insurance should be tied to the applicant's BMI. Smokers pay more for premiums because their care costs more. We believe the same should be true for an elevated BMI.

We have a few further suggestions of policy changes in several areas that could reduce the prevalence of obesity:[27]

Education

- Require instruction in nutrition and weight management as part of the school curriculum for future health-education teachers.
- Promote the annual National No-TV Week.
- Develop culturally relevant obesity prevention campaigns for high-risk and low-income American children.

Food Labeling and Advertising

- Require that containers for soft drinks and snacks sold in movie theaters, convenience stores, and other venues bear information about caloric, fat, trans fat, and sugar content.
- Require print advertisements to disclose the caloric content of the foods being marketed.

Food Assistance Programs

- Develop an incentive system to encourage food stamp recipients to purchase fruits, vegetables, whole grains, and other healthful foods.

Health Care and Training

- Require medical, nursing, and other health professions' curricula to teach the principles and benefits of healthful diet and exercise patterns.
- Require health care providers to learn about behavioral risks for obesity and how to counsel patients about health-promoting behavior change.
- Revise Medicaid and Medicare regulations to provide incentives to health care providers for nutrition and obesity counseling and other interventions that meet specified standards of cost and effectiveness.

Taxes

- Subsidize the costs of low-calorie, nutritious foods, perhaps by raising the costs of selected high-calorie, low-nutrient foods (yes, we favor a "fat tax").
- Remove sales taxes on, or provide other incentives for, purchase of exercise equipment.

Last, but not least, we join others in calling for the Centers for Disease Control and Prevention to become the nation's "command and control center" to manage the problem of childhood obesity. As should now be clear, we need an aggressive, coordinated national strategy. A single agency in charge of the problem of childhood obesity would, we believe, more effectively coordinate programs between state and federal agencies.

A 2004 report by a national health advocacy group, the Trust for America's Health, made several suggestions to the CDC with which we concur:[28]

- Coordinate all public education campaigns, including ones for kids.
- Establish national nutritional guidelines for the Food Guide Pyramid and National School Lunch Program based on health

research. This would take authority away from the U.S. Department of Agriculture so it can concentrate on its core mission of promoting the well-being of agriculture.

- Conduct a youth fitness study to evaluate school physical education programs and the impact of fitness on classroom performance.

- Be ready to react quickly and decisively when the Institute of Medicine, through the Food and Nutrition Board and the Board on Children, Youth, and Families, releases its comprehensive study of the science-based effects of food marketing on the diets and health of children and youth in the United States. This study is being funded by the Centers for Disease Control and Prevention in response to a congressional directive.[29]

WHAT CAN SCIENCE DO?

Periodically we hear on the nightly news or read in a newspaper or in a newsmagazine some breathless report of a promising miracle drug that could make obesity a thing of the past. In September 2004, for example, shares of Nastech Pharmaceutical soared 70 percent after the company announced an alliance with drug giant Merck to develop an appetite-regulating treatment for obesity.[30]

Some people hear news like this and think, *Why, that's wonderful! We can continue to eat like we have been, sit around all we want, and just take a pill to get slim! I like it!* But things seldom, if ever, work out that way in the real world.

"We shouldn't think there's going to be a magic pill out there," warned Peter Corr, senior vice president for science and technology at Pfizer, another drug giant. Right now Pfizer is studying more than forty molecular targets associated with weight gain, is testing two medicines in people, and has several others in various stages of animal studies.[31]

Make no mistake: Some intriguing discoveries are being made. Harvard University researchers, for example, recently discovered an

---

Food for Thought

"I strongly believe lifestyle changes should be the foundation of what we do. I would not want to see patients turn to a pill as the first approach."[33]

Dr. Sidney Smith
University of North Carolina

---

enzyme in the brain that monitors energy in cells and appears to regulate appetite and weight. When the scientists reduced the amount of the enzyme in mice, the animals ate less and lost weight. The opposite occurred when the mice got more of the enzyme. Any drug based on their research, however, is still years away.

An Associated Press report in March 2004 described a pill in development that appears to double the success rate of those who want to quit smoking, even as it helps them lose significant amounts of weight. "This is good news. The drug shows promise," declared Dr. Sidney Smith, cardiovascular chief at the University of North Carolina. But he quickly added, "However, I strongly believe lifestyle changes should be the foundation of what we do. I would not want to see patients turn to a pill as the first approach."[32]

We agree with Dr. Smith; while we welcome exciting new discoveries like these, we wouldn't want anyone to wait around for a magic pill in the hopes that it might solve all their health problems. And we have to remind ourselves, too, that we've often been disappointed by what turned out to be exaggerated claims. In 2002, for example, British scientists announced that they had developed a wonder drug that could potentially cure obesity. Their discovery, they said, could help to cut food intake by a third. Headlines around the world trumpeted the news, and at least two drug companies spent millions of dollars in experiments on the drug.

Two years later more than forty scientists from fifteen international research centers reported that they could not duplicate the British results, thus calling into question the value of the "discovery." They even took the unusual step of writing to the journal *Nature*—the

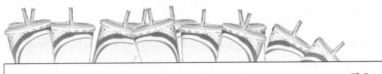

Fifty Ways to SuperSize Your Kids   #50

Believe that you can't make a difference when it comes to your child's health.

magazine that published the original claims—to express their disappointment. "For a moment," said researcher Matthias Tschop of the University of Cincinnati, "it seemed like we had a magic bullet for all patients." And yet when neither Tschop nor his colleagues could

Food for Thought

"We have a lot of work ahead of us."

Dr. George Blackburn
Harvard Medical School

duplicate the results claimed by the Brits, that bullet began to look more imaginary than magical.[34]

Don't waste your time waiting around for a magic pill to cure obesity. It probably isn't coming, and even if it did, it wouldn't cure all the serious ills associated with poor eating and too little exercise.

But if you're really interested in finding out about legislation in your state that promotes and supports healthy eating and physical activity, you can find a database of your state's physical activity and nutrition legislation on our Web site, www.SuperSizedKids.com, compiled by the National Conference of State Legislatures. A second database compiled by the CDC's Division of Nutrition and Physical Activity is also available.

LET'S GET STARTED

"We have a lot of work ahead of us," says George Blackburn, associate director of the division of nutrition at Harvard Medical School.[35]

How right he is! There is much work to be done, by all of us. But parents stand in the ideal position to get this work started. And what matters most now is that you begin this work by becoming your child's health care quarterback.

Start by making one or two small changes, from the hundreds we have suggested throughout this book. To help you with this, we have designed an eight-week plan for you and your family, found in Appendix B at the back of this book.

But don't stop there!

Keep the work going by getting involved with your community to create neighborhoods and schools that can become havens from obesity for America's children. And don't shrink from contacting your state senator or representative about issues that will make a difference in this crucial work.

You really can make a difference by taking that first small step. If we all work together, we can reverse the rising tide of childhood obesity and help to shrink our SuperSized Kids. United, we truly can take America's children from fat to fit.

Epilogue

A GOOD-NEWS ENDING

So very often it seems that happy endings occur only in fiction. But we have some good news for you! Happy endings can also happen in real life.

Remember Robert, the eleven-year-old we met in the first chapter who didn't like taking off his shirt at the pool because of the extra pounds he carried around? Sherri heard from his mother recently. And did the conversation ever put a smile on her face!

Robert has lost an additional ten pounds since we first met him. He has been handling school lunches by choosing fruits, veggies, and healthful-protein foods and staying away from the highly refined, high-sugar items. His mother also sends him to school with bottled water.

He stays active by walking, biking, and playing basketball with his friends and has a lot of fun in the process. He still watches some TV and plays some video games, but his mom says that many times he chooses to go outside and play instead.

Robert now goes grocery shopping with his mother (she laughed when she reported this) and reads almost every food label, looking especially for the sugar content. He is currently going through a growth spurt and seems to be hungry all the time—his mom gives him nuts as snacks and tries to stick with other healthy foods.

Robert recently had an appointment with his physician, who seemed very surprised at his weight loss. "No other family has ever taken me seriously when I said a child had to lose weight!" the doctor exclaimed. He told Robert that even if he maintained his current weight, chances were good because of his recent growth spurt that he would grow into his weight. Robert had to feel a great sense of accomplishment when he heard *that* news!

How did such a good-news story come about? It happened when Robert's doctor first told him about his prediabetic condition and how it could significantly harm his health. The boy took the physician's words seriously and, with his parents' direction, did something about it. His blood sugar levels are due to be tested again in a few months, but the physician expresses confidence that they will have dropped, due to the changes Robert and his family have made.

A great report like this does our hearts a lot of good. But you know what? It did Robert's heart a lot better. The same is true for each of the success stories we've experienced in our practices. Do you remember the stories we've told you of Hershel (Chapter 4), Tom (Chapter 4), John (Chapter 5), Betsy (Chapter 6), and Norman (Chapter 7)? In each case a SuperSized Kid and family made small decisions that resulted in large changes. Each family faced the perfect storm of childhood obesity—and each family won the battle.

There's no reason that something just as good couldn't happen in your own family.

But you'll need to decide to start. You'll have to get past the wishing and beyond the hoping. You'll have to put aside the resolutions and become resolute. You'll need to begin; you'll need to start.

For our part, we'll be working to assist schools, communities, and governments to come to your aid, to begin making the systemic changes that we hope will make your job easier and more successful.

It's going to take all of us—parents and families, physicians and health care providers, hospitals and insurance companies, school systems and communities, and your local, state, and federal government, all working together—to erase the scourge of SuperSized Kids from our land.

The perfect storm is brewing. But we pray and hope that by working together we can stem the threat.

Why don't we start together? Why don't we start today? Use the information you've learned and the tools we've provided to protect your kids—and their kids, and their kids' kids—from the threat of being SuperSized.

And when you do, you and your family will be that much closer to enjoying your own happy ending.

Appendix A

A THIRTY-MINUTE ASSESSMENT OF YOUR CHILD'S SUPERSIZE STATUS

This questionnaire has been designed not only to help you assess the degree of SuperSize risk your child or teen may face but also to introduce you to the factors you and your family can control to dramatically reduce this risk. We hope that by completing this questionnaire, you will gain a useful and instant snapshot of your child's SuperSize status.

This entire tool is available on the Internet in an easy-to-use, interactive form at www.SuperSizedKids.com. If you do not have access to the Internet, then we suggest that you photocopy the questionnaire's answer sheet (page 260). Use one answer sheet for each child in your family and let older children fill in their own forms. It might be fun for you and your spouse to complete the questionnaire as well. Then compare your findings and discuss them as a family.

Please note that this exercise is *not* meant for you to show your children where they come up short. Rather, this survey is designed to show where *you and your entire family* may need to improve in your quest to become healthier.

The more accurately you assess your child, the more helpful this tool will be. Although this measurement tool has not been scientifically tested, it is based upon our experience and an extensive review of the research literature.

As you read each description below, mark the appropriate answer to represent your evaluation of your child's SuperSize status.

NUTRITIONAL (10 QUESTIONS)

1. Vegetables

This section allows you to evaluate the average number of half-cup servings of vegetables that your child eats each day. Vegetables include, but are not limited to, artichokes, asparagus, bok choy, broccoli, brussels sprouts, cabbage, carrots, cauliflower, cucumbers, green beans, lettuce, mushrooms, mustard greens, onions, peas, peppers, potatoes, pumpkin, radish, salsa, spinach, squash, sweet potatoes, tomatoes, turnip greens, and zucchini. Do not include fries in your count.

5 points: 5 servings per day of veggies
4 points: 4 servings per day of veggies
3 points: 3 servings per day of veggies
2 points: 2 servings per day of veggies
1 point: 1 serving per day of veggies
0 points: no servings of veggies

2. Protein

For this section, you'll need to estimate your child's average daily intake of protein over the past three to four months. Lean meats, fish, lean poultry (chicken or turkey that is not fried), nuts (including peanut butter that does not contain trans fats), legumes, and eggs are all high-quality protein. Meats low in saturated fats, such as light-meat poultry without the skin (grilled or broiled), can add good protein to your child's diet with a minimum of bad fat. If your child is a vegetarian, he or she can get adequate protein from nonmeat sources. Do not count any fried foods in this category (such as fried fish or fried chicken).

5 points: more than 3 servings per day of good protein
3 points: 3 servings per day of good protein
2 points: 2 servings per day of good protein
1 point: 1 serving per day of good protein
0 points: no servings of good protein

3. Whole Grains

This section allows you to evaluate the average number of servings of whole grains your child eats each day. Healthy whole grain foods such as whole wheat, brown rice, and oatmeal are good sources of fiber, minerals, and some vitamins. Whole grain cereals or snack bars with minimal sugar content can be good breakfast choices for children. Stone-ground whole grains are also excellent and can be found at most grocery stores.

5 points: 3 or more servings per day of whole grains
3 points: 2 servings per day of whole grains
1 point: 1 serving per day of whole grains
0 points: no servings of whole grains

4. Fruits

This section allows you to evaluate the average number of half-cup or whole-piece servings of fruits your child eats each day. Fruits are incredibly healthy for children, packed as they are with fiber, water, vitamins, minerals, and antioxidants. Healthy fruits include, but are not limited to, apples, berries, cantaloupe, currants, grapefruit, grapes, honeydew, kiwifruit, kumquats, mangoes, nectarines, oranges, papayas, peaches, pineapple, plums, prunes, rhubarb, tangerines, strawberries, and watermelon. (A 6-ounce serving of 100 percent fruit juice equals one fruit serving—but don't count fruit juice on this question.)

5 points: 4 or more servings per day of fruit
3 points: 3 servings per day of fruit
2 points: 2 servings per day of fruit
1 point: 1 serving per day of fruit
0 points: no servings of fruit

5. Dairy and Calcium

This section allows you to evaluate either the average number of servings of calcium-containing foods (nonfat yogurt, nonfat milk, low-fat cheeses, soy-based products, whole grains, legumes, and calcium-fortified orange juice) or the calcium supplements your child ingests each day. Children and adolescents who cannot or will not consume adequate amounts of calcium from dietary sources should use mineral or calcium supplements, since the amount of calcium needed by a child (800 mg per day for four- to eight-year-olds and 1,300 mg per day for nine- to eighteen-year-olds) cannot be obtained from the vast majority of multivitamins. Remember that calcium is best absorbed when taken with food and that the average child cannot absorb more than 300 to 500 mg of calcium at any one meal.

5 points: 3 or more servings or a calcium supplement taken at two or three meals a day
3 points: 2 servings or a calcium supplement with only one meal
1 point: 1 serving and no calcium supplement
0 points: no calcium-containing food and no calcium supplement

6. Fast Food

For this section, consider the number of times your child ate at a fast-food restaurant each month, on average, over the past three or four months. By the way, as we discussed in Chapter 9, if your child can go to a fast-food restaurant and order a highly healthy meal (say, a fruit salad or a turkey sandwich with a cup of water), then don't count that in this section. Likewise, if your child goes to "sit-down" restaurants and eats unhealthy meals there, then do count those on this question.

5 points: not at all
4 points: one or two times per month
3 points: two or three times per month
2 points: one time per week
1 point: two or three times per week
0 points: more than four times per week

7. Soft Drinks

Most parents know that soft drinks and sodas are not the best choice they can make for their children. Even diet soft drinks would come in a distant second to 100 percent fruit juice or water. The acids used to carbonate and flavor these beverages can damage your child's teeth and may even weaken their bones. Soft drinks lack any real nutritional content. For this section, estimate your child's intake of soft drinks and sodas.

5 points: doesn't or rarely drinks soft drinks or sodas
4 points: less than 6 ounces one to three days per week
3 points: less than 6 ounces per day
2 points: 6 to 12 ounces per day (12 ounces is the average-sized can of soda)
1 point: 13 to 24 ounces per day
0 points: more than 24 ounces per day

8. Water

Water plays an essential role in maintaining health. Younger people need *more* fluids than adults, for the simple reason that their bodies are still growing—and demanding the hydration found in plain water. Of all the drinks available to our children, it's impossible to improve on fresh, pure, cool water. Drinking water is one extremely good habit that should last for a lifetime. For this section, estimate how many times a day your child drinks water. And we'll count nonfat (skim) milk or tea without sugar as a "water equivalent." In addition, a serving of fruit counts as a "water equivalent" (from question 4).

> **5 points:** one 8-ounce cup of water (or water equivalent) eight times per day, six or seven days per week
>
> **4 points:** one 8-ounce cup of water (or water equivalent) four or five times per day, four or five days per week
>
> **3 points:** one 8-ounce cup of water (or water equivalent) three times per day, four to six days per week
>
> **2 points:** one 8-ounce cup of water (or water equivalent) two or three times per day, two to four days per week
>
> **1 point:** seldom drinks water (or water equivalent) at or between meals (less than two 8-ounce cups of water per day)
>
> **0 points:** rarely drinks water (or water equivalent)

9. Fruit Drinks

To be labeled as a fruit juice, the Food and Drug Administration mandates that a product be 100 percent fruit juice. Any beverage less than 100 percent fruit juice must list the percentage of the product that is not fruit juice, and the beverage must include a descriptive term, such as "drink," "beverage," or "cocktail." In general, juice drinks contain between 10 percent and 99 percent juice, and almost all add sweeteners. Excessive juice or fruit drink consumption may contribute to the development of obesity. One study found a link between fruit juice intake in excess of 12 ounces per day and obesity.[1] For this section, you need to evaluate two factors: (1) your child's intake of 100 percent fruit juice and (2) your child's intake of fruit "drinks," "beverages," or "cocktails." Record the lowest possible score on your answer sheet.

For children two to six years old:

5 points: 6 ounces or less per day of 100 percent fruit juice, *or* no fruit "drinks," "beverages," or "cocktails"

4 points: 7 to 12 ounces per day of 100 percent fruit juice, *or* fruit "drinks," "beverages," or "cocktails" no more than two days per week

3 points: 13 to 18 ounces per day of 100 percent fruit juice, *or* fruit "drinks," "beverages," or "cocktails" three or four days per week

2 points: 19 to 24 ounces per day of 100 percent fruit juice, *or* fruit "drinks," "beverages," or "cocktails" five days per week

1 point: more than 24 ounces per day of 100 percent fruit juice, *or* fruit "drinks," "beverages," or "cocktails" six days per week

0 points: fruit "drinks," "beverages," or "cocktails" seven days per week

For children seven to eighteen years old:

5 points: no more than 12 ounces per day of 100 percent fruit juice, *or* no fruit "drinks," "beverages," or "cocktails"

4 points: 13 to 18 ounces per day of 100 percent fruit juice, *or* fruit "drinks," "beverages," or "cocktails" no more than two days per week

3 points: 19 to 24 ounces per day of 100 percent fruit juice, *or* fruit "drinks," "beverages," or "cocktails" three or four days per week

2 points: 25 to 36 ounces per day of 100 percent fruit juice, *or* fruit "drinks," "beverages," or "cocktails" five days per week

1 point: more than 36 ounces per day of 100 percent fruit juice, *or*
fruit "drinks," "beverages," or "cocktails" six days per week
0 points: fruit "drinks," "beverages," or "cocktails" seven days per week

10. Sweets and Unhealthful Snacks

Many nutrition experts tell us that highly processed foods with high concentrations of simple sugars (sweets) should be eaten rarely, if at all. Most snack foods fall into this category. Sweets and many snack foods contain "empty calories" that may contribute to weight gain and risk for diabetes. For this section, don't count soft drinks or sugar-containing fruit drinks. Think more in terms of solid or frozen sweets or dessert-type foods (cakes, pies, ice cream, candy bars, chips, cookies, etc.). Once again, think of your child's average intake over the past three to four months.

5 points: less than 1 serving per week
4 points: 1 small serving one or two times per week
3 points: 1 small serving three or four times per week
2 points: 1 small serving five or six times per week
1 point: 1 small serving seven times per week
0 points: large servings of sweets on some days, *or* sweets more than once a day

ACTIVITY (10 QUESTIONS)

11. Activity with Moderate Exertion

For children of elementary school age, activities with moderate exertion should be age-appropriate and developmentally appropriate. These activities should include a variety, such as running, playing on playground equipment, hide-and-seek, soccer, etc. For middle and high school children, moderate exercise would include a combination of (a) aerobic exercise, such as swimming, biking, or brisk walking, and (b) recreational sports, such as basketball, soccer, tennis, or hiking. For this and the next section, the minutes do not have to be consecutive—but the more days a week, the better. Three 20-minute activities count the same as one 60-minute activity.

5 points: 60 or more minutes per day, five to seven days per week (more than 300 minutes per week)

4 points: 60 or more minutes per day, four or five days per week (240 to 300 minutes per week)

3 points: 30 minutes per day, six or seven days per week, *or* 60 minutes per day, four or five days per week (180 to 240 minutes per week)

2 points: 15 minutes per day, four to seven days per week, *or* up to 30 minutes per day, two to six days per week (60 to 180 minutes per week)

1 point: 10 minutes per day, three to six days per week, *or* up to 20 minutes per day, two or three days per week (30 to 60 minutes per week)

0 points: less than 30 minutes per week

12. Activity with Little Exertion

To measure this section, consider your child's less exertional exercise (such as walking, playing, or yard work, or less energetic sports, such as bowling, golf, or softball). All things being equal, the health benefits of these types of activities will be greater if they're done with family members or friends.

5 points: at least 30 minutes, six or seven times per week, with other family members or friends (more than 180 minutes per week)

4 points: at least 30 minutes, four or five times per week, with other family members or friends (120 to 180 minutes per week), *or* at least 30 minutes alone, six to seven times per week (more than 180 minutes per week)

3 points: at least 30 minutes, two to four times per week, with other family members or friends (60 to 120 minutes per week), *or* at least 30 minutes alone, four or five times per week (120 to 180 minutes per week)

2 points: at least 30 minutes, one or two times per week, with other family members or friends (30 to 60 minutes per week), *or* at least 30 minutes alone, three or four times per week (90 to 120 minutes per week)

1 point: 15 to 30 minutes alone, one to three times per week (15 to 90 minutes per week)

0 points: not at all

13. Daily Movement with Minimal Exertion

This section estimates your child's "everyday activity" over the past three to four months (such as walking the dog, taking several flights of stairs, parking farther away from a building and walking, walking or biking to school or a friend's house instead of riding in a car, etc.). In other words, how often does your child consciously choose activity over convenience?

5 points: always (activity seven days a week)
4 points: often (activity six days a week)
3 points: sometimes (activity five days a week)
2 points: infrequently (activity three or four days a week)
1 point: rarely (activity one or two days a week)
0 points: never (my child is sedentary—a couch potato)

14. Adequate Rest

On average, over the past two to three months, how would you assess your child's sleep and rest habits? Consider these factors for this section:

1. My child goes to bed at a reasonable hour.
2. My child gets nine or more hours of restful sleep most nights of the week.
3. My child usually wakes up refreshed.
4. My child has downtime or quiet time every day.
5. My child enjoys one or more adequate, restful family vacations each year.

5 points: My child achieves five of the above.
4 points: My child achieves four of the above.
3 points: My child achieves three of the above.
2 points: My child achieves two of the above.
1 point: My child achieves one of the above.
0 points: My child achieves none of the above.

15. Extracurricular Activities

For this section, count your child's extracurricular activities (team sports, hobby groups, music lessons, dance lessons, cheerleading, clubs, scouting, youth groups, etc.) that meet at least weekly.

5 points: one or two extracurricular activities
4 points: three extracurricular activities
3 points: four extracurricular activities
2 points: five extracurricular activities
1 point: six or more extracurricular activities or *no* extracurricular activities
0 points: seven or more extracurricular activities

16. Family Meals at Home

For this section, we look at the number of meals per week, on average, over the past three to four months in which your family (parents and the child you're rating) sat down to share a meal together at home.

5 points: more than five meals per week
4 points: four meals per week
3 points: three meals per week
2 points: two meals per week
1 point: one meal per week
0 points: no meals as a family in the average week

17. TV/Internet/Video Games

The more time a child spends with the TV, the Internet, or playing video/computer games, the more likely he or she is to be SuperSized. Kids of healthier weight tend to have parents who know how to set limits when it comes to media. Where does your child line up? Remember to think in terms of your child's average media activity over the past three to four months.

5 points: Our home is TV free. The computer/Internet is used only in a public area of our home and only for educational purposes. I monitor what my child does on the Internet.

4 points: My child watches one hour or less a day, and the computer/Internet is used only in a public area of our home and for educational purposes. If my child watches TV, I routinely monitor what he or she watches. I monitor what my child does on the Internet.

3 points: My child is routinely exposed to one to two hours a day of media (television, videos, video games, and computer activities). I sometimes monitor what my child watches on TV and does on the Internet.

2 points: My child is routinely exposed to two to three hours a day of media, *or* it is unusual for me to monitor what my child watches on TV and does on the Internet.

1 point: My child is routinely exposed to three to four hours a day of media, *or* I rarely monitor what my child watches on TV and does on the Internet.

0 points: My child is routinely exposed to four or more hours a day of media, *or* I never monitor what my child watches on TV or does on the Internet.

Subtract 1 point if your child has a TV in his or her bedroom and subtract another point for Internet access in the bedroom.

18. Eating Away from Home

For the meals your child eats away from home, whether at the school lunchroom, friends' homes, or restaurants, what percent of those consist of mostly healthful choices—for example, includes fruits and vegetables or whole grains; water or nonfat dairy; lean meat, fish, or legumes—while avoiding sodas, sweets, fried food (burgers, chicken, fries), fat-filled salad dressings or sauces?

5 points: always (90 to 100 percent)
4 points: most of the time (80 to 90 percent)
3 points: often (70 to 80 percent)
2 points: sometimes (50 to 70 percent)
1 point: infrequently (25 to 50 percent)
0 points: rarely (less than 25 percent)

19. Serving Habits

For this section, consider the following factors:

1. I let my children who are old enough serve their own plates most, if not all, of the time.
2. I use small or medium-sized plates for meals, not the large dinner plates.
3. We have at least two courses with most dinners—for example, a small salad and then the main course.
4. I don't make my children clean their plates.
5. I don't use food as a reward for my children.

6. My children who are old enough help with the meal preparation and with cleanup after the meal.

7. If the phone rings during family mealtimes, we usually let it
ring.

8. My spouse and I usually or always resist the urge to fuss or lecture our children during family mealtimes.

5 points: Our family achieves seven or eight of the above.

4 points: Our family achieves five or six of the above.

3 points: Our family achieves three or four of the above.

2 points: Our family achieves two of the above.

1 point: Our family achieves one of the above.

0 points: Our family achieves none of the above.

20. Eating with the TV On

Use this section to measure the average number of meals per week,
over the past three to four months, in which your child ate a meal or
snacked in front of the TV. Be sure to include in this number meals
that were eaten while the TV was on, even if you ate at the dinner
table.

5 points: no meals or snacks in front of the TV or with the TV on

4 points: one meal or snack in front of the TV or with the TV on

3 points: two meals or snacks in front of the TV or with the TV on

2 points: three meals or snacks in front of the TV or with the
TV on

1 point: four meals or snacks in front of the TV or with the TV on

0 points: five or more meals or snacks in front of the TV or with
the TV on, *or* my child virtually always has the TV on
when he or she eats or snacks at home.

FAMILY BMI (4 QUESTIONS)

As we near the finish line, let's turn our attention to one last section: the SuperSize Family History. This section will not determine any points for your child's SuperSize score but will provide a rough measure of your family's SuperSize health, at least as based upon the body mass index (BMI) of each member of your family. The American Academy of Pediatrics now recommends that all children over age two be assessed for growth by using their BMI instead of using the older height and weight charts.

21. Child's BMI

For this section, you'll need to determine your child's body mass index (BMI). You can determine your child's BMI on our Internet site (www.SuperSize.com) or by using the chart in Appendix C. To do this, you'll need your child's exact height, weight, and age. The BMI, when applied to children aged two through twenty, is expressed in a term called percentile. The Centers for Disease Control avoids using the word "obesity" to refer to children and adolescents. Instead, it suggests two levels of overweight: (1) the 85th percentile, an "at risk" level, and (2) the 95th percentile, the more severe level. The American Obesity Association, however, uses the 85th percentile of BMI as a reference point for overweight and the 95th percentile for obesity. For our purposes, we'll use the terminology and definitions of the American Obesity Association.[2]

Since body mass index doesn't directly measure body fat, an abnormal BMI doesn't necessarily mean your child is overweight or obese. Some very athletic kids who have a large muscle mass may have a high BMI; but if they do not have excess body fat, then they do not need help with weight loss. The vast majority of children with elevated BMIs, however, are overweight and do need help with weight management.

In addition, being underweight or at risk of being underweight means that your child has a body mass index for his or her age lower than the 15th percentile. This can be normal, especially if your child has been growing and developing normally, has a nutritious diet, and is active and energetic. Being underweight, however, can also signal a problem and deserves a full medical exam.

Determine your child's score by using these criteria:

5 points: BMI 16th to 84th percentile (normal BMI)
3 points: BMI 6th to 15th percentile (at risk for being under-weight) or 85th to 94th percentile (overweight)
1 point: BMI 5th percentile or less (underweight) or at or above the 95th percentile (obese)

22. Siblings' BMI

For the next score, determine the BMI percentile of each of your child's siblings (whether natural or adopted) who live with you and your child. Add up these BMIs and then divide by the number of the children to determine the average BMI of the siblings of the child you are evaluating. For example, if your child has three siblings, one with a BMI of the 85th percentile, one with a BMI of the 90th percentile, and one with a BMI above the 95th percentile, their total BMI percentile would be 270 (85 + 90 + 95). Divide this number by 3 (the number of siblings) to arrive at the average sibling BMI percentile of 90. This would result in 3 points, using these criteria:

5 points: BMI 16th to 84th percentile (normal BMI)
3 points: BMI 6th to 15th percentile (at risk for being under-weight) or 85th to 94th percentile (overweight)
1 point: BMI 5th percentile or less (underweight) or at or above the 95th percentile (obese)

23. and 24. Father's and Mother's BMI

For these, determine the BMI of the child's mother and father who live with the child. You can determine your BMI on our Internet site (www.SuperSize.com) or by using the BMI table in Appendix C. For adults, use just the BMI (not a percentile).

If the mother or the father is a stepparent, then use the stepparent's BMI and not the natural parent's BMI (as the stepparent will, we believe, have more influence on the child's nutrition and activity than the natural parent's genetics). If the child lives in your home and you and your spouse are raising the child (and are not the child's parent), then use your BMI. If you are a single person raising the child, then use your BMI and estimate the BMI of the missing natural parent. If the missing parent(s) is (are) unknown to you, then use your BMI for both ratings.

Use these criteria for the score:

5 points: BMI 18.5 to 25.9 (healthy weight)
3 points: BMI of 25 to 26.9 (mildly to moderately overweight)
2 points: BMI of 27 to 29.9 (moderately to severely overweight)
1 point: BMI of 30 to 39.9 (obese)
0 points: BMI of 40 or more (massive or morbid obesity), or BMI less than 18.5 (underweight)

Thirty-Minute Assessment Answer Sheet

Nutrition Section	Activity Section	Family BMI
1) ___	11) ___	21) ___
2) ___	12) ___	22) ___
3) ___	13) ___	23) ___
4) ___	14) ___	24) ___
5) ___	15) ___	
6) ___	16) ___	
7) ___	17) ___	
8) ___	18) ___	
9) ___	19) ___	
10) ___	20) ___	

TOTAL NUTRITION SCORE (add up the points in 1 to 10 and multiply by 2) = ___

TOTAL ACTIVITY SCORE (add up the points in 11 to 20 and multiply by 2) = ___

TOTAL FAMILY BMI SCORE (add up the points in 21 to 24 and multiply by 5) = ___

Now give your child a grade based upon each of these scores:

A = 90–100
B = 80–89
C = 70–79
D = 60–69
F = Below 60

NUTRITION GRADE   = ___

ACTIVITY GRADE   = ___

FAMILY BMI GRADE   = ___

WHAT DO I DO NOW?

Now that you've finished and graded the assessment for your child(ren), you'll be able to plan a strategy to improve your child's SuperSize grades. Reading this book will equip you to do just that. If you take these principles to heart and apply them, you'll see the scores and grades improve as you make the decisions necessary to nurture children who will not become SuperSized.

1. Identify the questions in the Nutritional and Activity sections that have the lowest scores and then concentrate on these issues. If your child has more than one area with equally low scores (for example, if three of the questions have only 2 points), choose the one you consider the easiest to address, and reread the section of the book that highlights that area.

And if several (or many) of the questions have equally low scores, choose the *one* you consider the *easiest* to fix, and reread the section of the book that deals with that area. In the table on the next page, you can find the section of the book addressing each question. After you know more about this area of health, go to step 2 below.

2. Once you've completed the assessment and educated yourself on some of the basics, turn to our eight-week plan on page 265 and familiarize yourself with the options available for your family.

3. Now it's time to get started taking some small, simple steps that will result in big results for you and your children. It's time to decide upon your family's individual action plan. We recommend that you hold a family meeting to discuss the problems you've found and the possible actions you could take as a family. As you discuss some of these ideas with your spouse and children, which do they like? Which would they be willing to try? Do you or they have additional ideas about steps you could take that we haven't mentioned? Remember, small changes can result in big health benefits. Don't be surprised if it

takes two or three family meetings to come up with a plan that the
entire family will agree upon.

Nutrition		Activity	
Nutritional question 1	Chapter 9, pages 132–134	Activity question 11	Chapter 8, pages 112–131
Nutritional question 2	Chapter 9, pages 134–135	Activity question 12	Chapter 8, pages 112–130
Nutritional question 3	Chapter 9, pages 135–138	Activity question 13	Chapter 8, pages 112–130
Nutritional question 4	Chapter 9, pages 132–134	Activity question 14	Chapter 6, pages 80–92
Nutritional question 5	Chapter 9, pages 138–141	Activity question 15	Chapter 8, pages 112–130
Nutritional question 6	Chapter 9, pages 150–151	Activity question 16	Chapter 10, pages 170–174
Nutritional question 7	Chapter 9, pages 146–149	Activity question 17	Chapter 7, pages 93–111
Nutritional question 8	Chapter 9, pages 148	Activity question 18	Chapter 3, pages 31–32
Nutritional question 9	Chapter 9, pages 146–149	Activity question 19	Chapter 10, pages 162–165
Nutritional question 10	Chapter 10, pages 174–176	Activity question 20	Chapter 7, pages 100–101

4. Once you have a plan, it's time to get started! Are you willing
to take the necessary actions to help your children avert or reverse
being SuperSized? You may have to ask for advice from trusted health
care providers or a registered dietitian. It will take some time, but the
simple steps we outline in this book do work!

5. Keep making progress. Once you've fixed the area you've cho-
sen to address, reassess your child's SuperSize score and then choose

another area to address. And even if your child is scoring an A, consider checking your child's SuperSize score by retaking the assessment test every six to twelve months.

Let us be perfectly clear. *This is going to involve work.* But we've already shown how you can do it, and do it successfully.

At times, you or your child may feel tempted to stop halfway down the road. But let us reassure you that the hard work and effort will be worth it. The sacrifice of time and effort won't be wasted. Your effort can and will greatly benefit the generations to come.

Appendix B

AN EIGHT-WEEK PLAN: REDUCE THE SUPERSIZE THREAT TO YOUR FAMILY

Are you ready to start? Are you looking forward to taking some small steps toward reducing the threat of obesity in your home and, at the same time, making your family more healthy?

We've taken many of the tips contained in this book and arranged them into our eight-week plan for reducing the SuperSize threat to your family. Each week in the plan will take a little bit more work and effort, building on what you've done the previous week, but all of the steps are simple—they just require a little determination. And we guarantee that the rewards will make it more than worth it!

We suggest you first read over these steps. Then set a time to begin. The holiday season or the first week of the school year may not be a good time to start (as there is so much going on), but summertime or a week or two after the start of school can be a great time to begin.

We know some of you will be ready to jump right in and do all the steps we've suggested for each week. That's wonderful! But it's okay if you feel this would be too dramatic or too quick for your family. No problem at all—just slow it down. Pick one step each week in each category, or every other week, or even one step a month. That way, you'll be at the end of the plan in either four or eight months—but either way, your family will be healthier. Finishing at your own pace is more important than starting and not finishing!

Beware that doing too much too quickly can also be harmful. If you go at this program with too much intensity, there might be a backlash from your family. You'll need to be sensitive to the family relationships in order to have the greatest success. For example, if you try to alter your child's habit pattern too quickly or change multiple habits at once, there will be a negative response unless you include the child in the process and make it something fun for the whole family.

If you or your child gets sore or injured from the new exercise program, you or the child are likely to quit the program entirely. The answer are moderation and gradual steady changes in lifestyle that the body, mind, and spirit will tolerate. Everyone will be happier (and healthier) as a result.

You might want to photocopy each week's plan from the book and post it on the refrigerator or on a family bulletin board, to easily refer to during the week. You can even highlight the goals you want to focus on as a family. At the end of each week, have a family meeting to assess your progress. Be sure to listen to and value the input from the children, but always remember that you are the gatekeeper as well as quarterback and give them reasonable answers to their questions.

Remember that kids love rewards, affirmation, and positive feedback. We've developed certificates of achievement that you can adapt for your child and print off from our Web site at www.SuperSized-Kids.com. You can present your child with a diploma each week of the plan.

At the end of the eight-week program, have a summary family meeting. Discuss which steps worked well for your family and which did not. Decide which ones you want to permanently incorporate into your family health plan. In just eight weeks not only will you have created a foundation that will give great rewards to you and your family, but we bet you'll be ready to look for other ways you can become even healthier.

Week 1

Family Project

- Get a blank notebook and start a family health journal to keep track of your progress.
- Use Appendix C to calculate the BMI (and blood pressure if possible) for each family member and record it in your journal.

Activities

- Take the blank activity pyramid on page 128 and talk about what you could do as a family. Record your ideas in your journal.
- See how many steps you and each child can climb or how far you can quickly walk without getting short of breath. Write it down in the journal.

Mealtimes at Home

- Use an answering machine during dinner at home.
- Reduce the visits to fast-food restaurants by one per week.
- Switch from large to small dinner plates.

Nutrition

- Eat at least one serving of fruit or vegetables at each meal.
- Strategize with your kids about how to increase their intake of plant protein. Try one of their ideas this week.

Rest

- Cut out the caffeine (chocolate, cocoa, soft drinks) after 3 P.M.

Media

- Cut your child's media time (total TV, computer, and video game time) to less than four hours a day.
- Remove the TV, computer, and video game machines from the bedrooms and move them to a common area.

Week 2

Family Project

- Have a family meeting to discuss the progress you made during the first week. What worked? What didn't? What was fun? What was unrewarding? What have you learned? What else do you want to change? Make notes in your journal.

- As a family, learn how to read food labels by studying items in your kitchen. (Refer to Chapter 9, especially page 145, for tips on label reading.)

- Plan to shop together for groceries once a month and be sure to review food labels at the store.

Activities

- Begin planning exercise for the week for each family member.

Mealtimes at Home

- Turn off the TV during meals.

- Reduce desserts to smaller portions and no more than one per day. Try replacing desserts with fresh fruit.

- Children who are old enough to do so can serve their own plates.

Nutrition

- Reduce red meat to no more than three meals a week.

- Begin trying new fish recipes or vegetarian protein recipes.

Rest

- Set and enforce bedtime and wake-up time (see page 87).

Media

- Try a TV-free night one day this week (or make it a media-free night).

Week 3

Family Project

- Have a family meeting to discuss the progress you made during the second week and record your progress.
- Reduce or eliminate foods with trans fats (hydrogenated or partially hydrogenated oils).

Activities

- Try to exercise as a family at least once this week.
- Review the progress of each family member regarding his/her individual activity each day.

Mealtimes at Home

- Discuss as a family how you could increase the number of family meals.
- Plan at least two courses for each meal, with five minutes between courses.

Nutrition

- If you are using whole milk, change to 2 percent. If you are using 2 percent, change to 1 percent.
- Start eating a serving of fish or lean poultry at least twice a week.
- Start eating a serving of plant protein (beans, nuts, soy, etc.) at least twice a week.

Rest

- Be sure all children are getting at least seven hours of sleep every night.

Media

- Cut media time to two hours or less a day.

Week 4

Family Project

- Have a family meeting to discuss and record the progress you made during the third week.
- Reduce the amount of sodas, fruit drinks, and other sugared drinks—consider cutting the number in half.
- Begin serving water with family meals (see page 148).

Activities

- Find and do a fun physical activity for the family for this weekend (we've got some suggestions on page 129).
- Retest the family to see how many steps each of you can climb or how far each of you can quickly walk without getting short of breath. Record your results and compare them to week 1. How much progress have you made?

Mealtimes at Home

- Plan to eat together as a family at least three meals a week.
- Reduce desserts to three meals a week.
- Work to make family meals fun.
- Don't fuss at family meals.
- Ask lots of questions of your kids at meals and then listen to their answers.

Nutrition

- Have at least two servings of fruits or vegetables at each meal.
- Reduce or eliminate fried foods.

Rest

- No TV or computer within one hour of bedtime.

Media

- Try a TV-free (or media-free) night two days this week.

Week 5

Family Project

- Have a family meeting to discuss and record the progress you made during the fourth week.
- Have healthful snacks available, especially for after school and weekends.

Activities

- Walk with your kids to school, if possible.
- Park farther away from stores and walk.

Mealtimes at Home

- Beginning this week, no snacking in front of the TV or computer.
- Begin watching and reducing portion sizes.

Nutrition

- Reduce red meat to no more than two meals a week.
- Increase your fish or lean poultry consumption to at least three times a week.
- Increase plant protein consumption to at least three times a week.

Rest

- Be sure all children are getting at least eight hours of sleep every night.

Media

- Cut media time to less than an hour a day.

Week 6

Family Project

- Have a family meeting to discuss and record the progress you made during the fifth week.

- Plan to shop for groceries together once every one or two weeks and be sure to review nutrition labels at the store. Plan plenty of time and have fun (see page 71)!

- Teach children how to compare prices and value. Calculate the cost per ounce, pound, etc., and determine which is the best dollar value for the nutrient impact.

- Reduce the amount of sodas, fruit drinks, and other sugared drinks—consider cutting the number in half (you might have done this once already in week 4).

Activities

- Try to exercise as a family at least twice this week.

- Review again the progress each of you is making in daily activity.

Mealtimes at Home

- Begin eating together as a family at least five meals a week.

- Reduce desserts to two a week.

- Look at the food pyramid and decide how you can improve your family food choices.

Nutrition

- If you are using 2 percent milk, change to 1 percent. If you are using 1 percent, change to skim milk.

- Be sure your kids are getting a serving of a healthful whole grain food once a day.

Rest

- Give kids a thirty-minute warning before bedtime.

Media

- Try a TV-free (or media-free) night three days this week.

Week 7

Family Project

- Have a family meeting to discuss and record the progress you made during the sixth week.

- Together with your kids, examine your pantry and refrigerator and choose the unhealthful foods you would like to get rid of. Then begin to eliminate them.

Activities

- Try to exercise as a family at least three times this week.

Mealtimes at Home

- Discuss as a family how everyone can begin having breakfast most days of the week (see page 164).

- Try to cut out all or most sweets.

- Begin using the blank food pyramid to plan a week's worth of family meals (see page 157).

Nutrition

- Reduce red meat to no more than one meal a week.

- Increase fish or lean poultry consumption to at least five times a week.

- Increase plant protein consumption to at least five times a week.

Rest

- Try to see that everyone in the family gets nine hours of sleep every night.

Media

- If you haven't already done so, now's the time to get the TV or Internet out of the child's bedroom.

Week 8

Family Project

- Recheck every family member's BMI and blood pressure and compare them to the values you obtained in week 1.
- Have a family meeting to review your eight-week journey.
- Consider evaluating each child in the family with the assessment tool in Appendix A.

Activities

- Meet as a family to talk about how far you've come these past two months and what you'd each like to do next.
- Discuss how regular physical activity will continue to be a part of the daily family routine.
- Test yourself and each child to see how many steps you can climb or how far you can quickly walk without getting short of breath. How much progress has each person made?
- Try to exercise as a family at least four times this week.

Mealtimes at Home

- Increase the times you eat together as a family to at least seven meals a week.
- Review with your family how you could continue to improve your nutrition at home.

Nutrition

- If you are using 1 percent milk, change to skim milk.
- Be sure your kids are getting three servings of a healthful whole grain food each day.
- Be sure that your kids are eating healthful protein two or three times a day.

Rest

- Talk as a family about how the "rest" experiments have worked. What do you want to continue? What do you want to change?

Media

- Try one week without any TV or computer.
- Plan a family night to discuss how you've done with media. What's worked? What has not?

Congratulations! You've finished the plan. We bet that when you first looked at it, you wondered if you could do it. Right? But now you've done it! Well done!

Remember, although you and your children have made some wise and life-changing decisions, this is just the beginning of the rest of your life. The decisions you've made and the steps you've taken have reduced your child's chance of obesity, diabetes, high blood pressure, arthritis, heart disease, stroke, cancer, and premature death. But now the work of continuing most or all of these steps lies before you.

What can your family do to become even more healthy?

If you've had difficulty with the weekly plan, or if these suggestions have not been helpful for your family, consider an appointment with a registered dietitian or a weight-loss center that has a program designed for children.

If you haven't already used the assessment tool in Appendix A, we suggest you do so at the end of the eight-week plan. It may show you other areas you can concentrate on to improve your child's and your family's health.

You can also check out www.SuperSizedKids.com or www.DrWalt .com for links to other helpful books and assessment tools. There you can explore ways you and your children can become more healthy, not only physically (building on all you learned in this book) but emotionally, relationally, and spiritually as well.

Know that as you continue this journey, you have our best wishes and prayers for a fruitful and satisfying trip down the highway of life.

Appendix C

BODY MASS INDEX (BMI)
FOR CHILDREN AND TEENS

BMI charts are used differently with children and teens than they are with adults. The normal body fatness of children and teens changes over the years as they grow. Also, girls and boys differ in their body fatness as they mature.

This is why the BMI-for-children and -teens, also referred to as BMI-for-age, is gender and age specific. BMI-for-age is plotted on gender specific growth charts. To evaluate your child or teen's SuperSize status, you'll need to follow two steps:

1. If you know your child's height (in inches) and weight (in pounds), you can find your child's BMI on the **BMI Table** on page 279. Or, you can use an Internet-based BMI calculator at our Web site www.SuperSizedKids.com.

2. Plot your child's BMI on one of the **BMI Percentile** graphs—there is one for girls (page 280) and one for boys (page 281). To use these graphs, find your child's **BMI** in the left-hand column. Then, move across the columns until you get to your child's **age** and make a mark on the graph at this point. You can then see which curved line is the closest to this point of the graph—and this curved line will tell your child's **BMI Percentile**.

You can use your child's BMI Percentile to determine if your child or teen is underweight, overweight, or obese. If your child's BMI-for-age is:

- **At or below the 5th percentile**, then your child is **underweight**.
- The **6th to 15th percentile**, then your child is **at risk of becoming underweight**.
- The **16th to 84th percentile**, then your child is **normal weight**. Congratulations!
- The **85th to 94th percentile**, then your child is **overweight**.
- **At or above the 95th percentile**, then your child is **obese**.

BMI Table for Children and Teens

To use the table on the next page, find your child's or teen's **height** in the left-hand column. Then, move across the row to your child's or teen's **weight**. The number at the top of the column is your child's or teen's BMI. We suggest you round pounds up and inches down.

Family Body Mass Index Table

BMI	13	14	15	16	17	18	19	20	21	22	23	24	25	26	27	28	29	30	31	32	33	34	35	36
Inches																								
33"	20	22	23	25	26	28	29	31	33	34	36	37	39	40	42	43	45	46	48	50	51	53	54	56
34"	21	23	25	26	28	30	31	33	35	36	38	39	41	43	44	46	48	49	51	53	54	56	58	59
35"	23	24	26	28	30	31	33	35	37	38	40	42	44	45	47	49	51	52	54	56	58	59	61	63
36"	24	26	28	29	31	33	35	37	39	41	42	44	46	48	50	52	53	55	57	59	61	63	65	66
37"	25	27	29	31	33	35	37	39	41	43	45	47	49	51	53	55	56	58	60	62	64	66	68	70
38"	27	29	31	33	35	37	39	41	43	45	47	49	51	53	55	58	60	62	64	66	68	70	72	74
39"	28	30	32	35	37	39	41	43	45	48	50	52	54	56	58	61	63	65	67	69	71	74	76	78
40"	30	32	34	36	39	41	43	46	48	50	52	55	57	59	61	64	66	68	71	73	75	77	80	82
41"	31	33	36	38	41	43	45	48	50	53	55	57	60	62	65	67	69	72	74	77	79	81	84	86
42"	33	35	38	40	43	45	48	50	53	55	58	60	63	65	68	70	73	75	78	80	83	85	88	90
43"	34	37	39	42	45	47	50	53	55	58	60	63	66	68	71	74	76	79	82	84	87	89	92	95
44"	36	39	41	44	47	50	52	55	58	61	63	66	69	72	74	77	80	83	85	88	91	94	96	99
45"	37	40	43	46	49	52	55	58	60	63	66	69	72	75	78	81	84	86	89	92	95	98	101	104
46"	39	42	45	48	51	54	57	60	63	66	69	72	75	78	81	84	87	90	93	96	99	102	105	108
47"	41	44	47	50	53	57	60	63	66	69	72	75	79	82	85	88	91	94	97	101	104	107	110	113
48"	43	46	49	52	56	59	62	66	69	72	75	79	82	85	88	92	95	98	102	105	108	111	115	118
49"	44	48	51	55	58	61	65	68	72	75	79	82	85	89	92	96	99	102	106	109	113	116	120	123
50"	46	50	53	57	60	64	68	71	75	78	82	85	89	92	96	100	103	107	110	114	117	121	124	128
51"	48	52	55	59	63	67	70	74	78	81	85	89	92	96	100	104	107	111	115	118	122	126	129	133
52"	50	54	58	62	65	69	73	77	81	85	88	92	96	100	104	108	112	115	119	123	127	131	135	138
53"	52	56	60	64	68	72	76	80	84	88	92	96	100	104	108	112	116	120	124	128	132	136	140	144
54"	54	58	62	66	71	75	79	83	87	91	95	100	104	108	112	116	120	124	129	133	137	141	145	149
55"	56	60	65	69	73	77	82	86	90	95	99	103	108	112	116	120	125	129	133	138	142	146	151	155
56"	58	62	67	71	76	80	85	89	94	98	103	107	112	116	120	125	129	134	138	143	147	152	156	161
57"	60	65	69	74	79	83	88	92	97	102	106	111	116	120	125	129	134	139	143	148	153	157	162	166
58"	62	67	72	77	81	86	91	96	100	105	110	115	120	124	129	134	139	144	148	153	158	163	167	172
59"	64	69	74	79	84	89	94	99	104	109	114	119	124	129	134	139	144	149	154	158	163	168	173	178
60"	67	72	77	82	87	92	97	102	108	113	118	123	128	133	138	143	149	154	159	164	169	174	179	184
61"	69	74	79	85	90	95	101	106	111	116	122	127	132	138	143	148	153	159	164	169	175	180	185	191
62"	71	77	82	87	93	98	104	109	115	120	126	131	137	142	148	153	159	164	170	175	180	186	191	197
63"	73	79	85	90	96	102	107	113	119	124	130	135	141	147	152	158	164	169	175	181	186	192	198	203
64"	76	82	87	93	99	105	111	117	122	128	134	140	146	151	157	163	169	175	181	186	192	198	204	210
65"	78	84	90	96	102	108	114	120	126	132	138	144	150	156	162	168	174	180	186	192	198	204	210	216
66"	81	87	93	99	105	112	118	124	130	136	143	149	155	161	167	173	180	186	192	198	204	211	217	223
67"	83	89	96	102	109	115	121	128	134	140	147	153	160	166	172	179	185	192	198	204	211	217	223	230
68"	86	92	99	105	112	118	125	132	138	145	151	158	164	171	178	184	191	197	204	210	217	224	230	237
69"	88	95	102	108	115	122	129	135	142	149	156	163	169	176	183	190	196	203	210	217	223	230	237	244
70"	91	98	105	112	118	125	132	139	146	153	160	167	174	181	188	195	202	209	216	223	230	237	244	251
71"	93	100	108	115	122	129	136	143	151	158	165	172	179	186	194	201	208	215	222	229	237	244	251	258
72"	96	103	111	118	125	133	140	147	155	162	170	177	184	192	199	206	214	221	229	236	243	251	258	265
73"	99	106	114	121	129	136	144	152	159	167	174	182	190	197	205	212	220	227	235	243	250	258	265	273
74"	101	109	117	125	132	140	148	156	164	171	179	187	195	203	210	218	226	234	241	249	257	265	273	280
75"	104	112	120	128	136	144	152	160	168	176	184	192	200	208	216	224	232	240	248	256	264	272	280	288
76"	107	115	123	131	140	148	156	164	173	181	189	197	205	214	222	230	238	246	255	263	271	279	288	296
77"	110	118	127	135	143	152	160	169	177	186	194	202	211	219	228	236	245	253	261	270	278	287	295	304

2 to 20 years: Girls
Body mass index-for-age percentiles

NAME _____

RECORD # _____

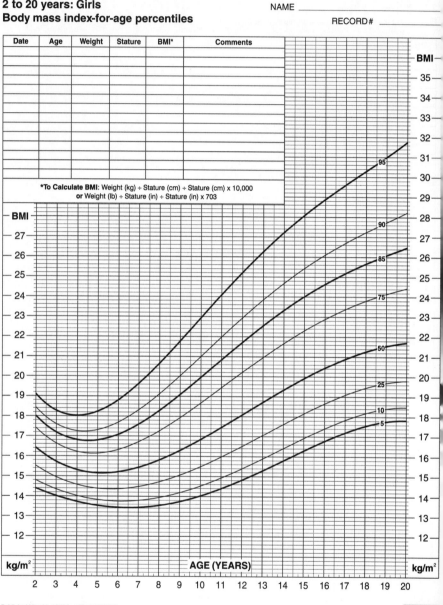

Date	Age	Weight	Stature	BMI*	Comments

*To Calculate BMI: Weight (kg) ÷ Stature (cm) ÷ Stature (cm) x 10,000
or Weight (lb) ÷ Stature (in) ÷ Stature (in) x 703

Published May 30, 2000 (modified 10/16/00).
SOURCE: Developed by the National Center for Health Statistics in collaboration with
the National Center for Chronic Disease Prevention and Health Promotion (2000).
http://www .cdc.gov/growthcharts

CDC

SAFER · HEALTHIER · PEOPLE

2 to 20 years: Boys
Body mass index-for-age percentiles

NAME

RECORD#

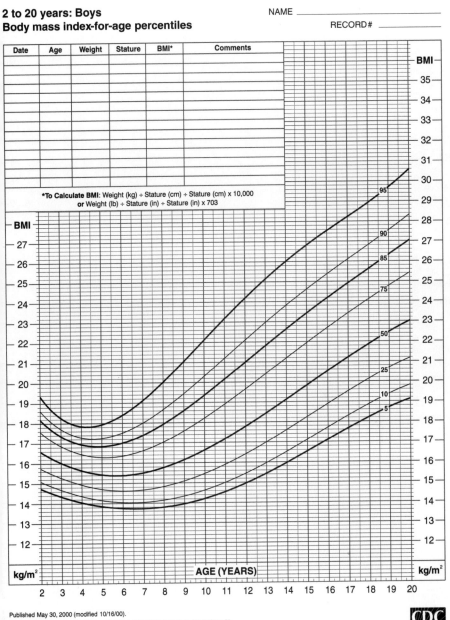

*To Calculate BMI: Weight (kg) ÷ Stature (cm) ÷ Stature (cm) x 10,000
or Weight (lb) ÷ Stature (in) ÷ Stature (in) x 703

AGE (YEARS)

Published May 30, 2000 (modified 10/16/00).

SOURCE: Developed by the National Center for Health Statistics in collaboration with
the National Center for Chronic Disease Prevention and Health Promotion (2000).
http://www .cdc.gov/growthcharts

CDC
SAFER·HEALTHIER·PEOPLE™

Appendix D

50 WAYS TO SUPERSIZE YOUR KIDS

1. Believe that your child's SuperSize status is normal.
2. SuperSize their portions!
3. Let your kids eat frequently at fast-food restaurants.
4. Give your kids lots of soft drinks!
5. Refuse to become your child's health care quarterback.
6. Consider your kid's SuperSize status *their* problem and not a *family* problem.
7. Fail to teach your kids good eating habits, especially when they are young.
8. Rarely eat together as a family.
9. Make impulsive decisions (or let your kids talk you into impulsive decisions) while grocery-shopping.
10. Don't involve your entire family in fun physical activity.
11. Let family or friends become diet saboteurs for your kids.
12. Keep your TV on during meals.
13. Let your children or teens sleep less than nine hours per night.
14. Let your kids have caffeinated drinks, cocoa, or chocolate after 3 P.M.
15. Let your kids go to bed as late as they want to. And let them watch TV right up until they go to bed.

16. Allow your kids to watch all the TV they want.

17. Permit your kids to eat or snack in front of the TV or keep the TV on during mealtime.

18. Give your child unrestricted TV and Internet access in his or her bedroom.

19. Allow your kids to play video games as much as they want to.

20. Never exercise with your kids.

21. Get some Elmer's and glue your kids to the couch.

22. Ignore fruits and vegetables in your children's diet.

23. Be sure your children get protein sources chock-full of saturated fats or ones that are fatty or fried.

24. Feed your kids plenty of highly processed, sugar-laden food.

25. Give your kids several servings each day of highly refined starches, such as white rice, white bread, potatoes without the skin, pasta, and baked goods.

26. Have your kids drink more soda than nonfat milk.

27. Insist that your kids eat or drink full-fat dairy products.

28. Give your kids snacks loaded with saturated and trans fats.

29. Choose fruit drinks instead of 100 percent fruit juice for your child.

30. Encourage your kids to drink anything but water.

31. Feed your kids crispy chicken or fried foods.

32. Use food as a reward for good behavior.

33. Make sure that your kids eat junk food or fast food every day.

34. Don't bother to learn the appropriate portion sizes for your child's age.

35. Let your child skip breakfast most days.

36. Buy your kids high-sugar, low-fiber, highly processed cereal and soak it with whole milk.

37. Don't bother with family meals; let everyone eat when they want.

38. Serve food to your children on large plates and then make them eat every bite.

39. Ban healthy snacks from your home.

40. Never plan ahead for your children's snacks.

41. Put your child on a diet.

42. Train your kids to eat as quickly as possible.

43. Support all moves to cut recess and physical education from your child's school.

44. Encourage your child's school to ignore healthy nutritional and activity habits.

45. Lobby your child's school to operate plenty of vending machines, stocked with lots of unhealthy foods and drinks.

46. Refuse to get informed about the nutritional and activity environment of your child's school.

47. Never volunteer or help out at your child's school.

48. Even if it's geographically possible, don't walk your children to school or let them walk to school.

49. Neglect good nutrition and physical activity where you work.

50. Believe that you can't make a difference when it comes to your child's health.

ENDNOTES

Chapter 1

1. The names (and occasionally the ages and/or sex) of all the children and patients mentioned in this book have been changed.

Chapter 2

1. "Study Finds Obesity Among New York City Children," Reuters Health, August 30, 2004.
2. "Many School Children Weigh Too Much," Reuters Health, June 3, 2004.
3. "U.S. Surgeon General Joins Nike, McNeil Nutritionals and American Academy of Pediatrics to Address National Trend of Childhood Inactivity and Unhealthy Diets," January 20, 2004, http://www.jnj.com/news/ jnj_news/20031103_100201.htm.
4. Shannon Brownlee, "Too Heavy, Too Young," *Time*, January 21, 2002, www.time.com/time/covers/1101020121/obesity.html.
5. Lindsey Tanner, "Study: We're Eating Ourselves to Death," Associated Press, March 9, 2004, http://member.compuserve.com/news/story.jsp? oldflock=FF-APO-1 . . .
6. "The Fairy Tale About Soft Drink Nutrition Won't Sell," editorial, *Boston Globe*, December 1, 2004, www.boston.com/news/globe/editorial_ opinion/oped/articles/2004/12/01/the_fairy_tale_about_sof.
7. "Obesity Gets Part of Blame for Care Costs," *Washington Post*, October 20, 2004, A03.
8. "Feds: Obesity Raising Airline Fuel Costs," Associated Press, November 5, 2004.
9. Dr. Gerald Hass, "Fast Food, Fat Kids," *Boston Globe*, December 23, 2002, http://www.commercialalert.org/obesityhass.htm.
10. Ibid.
11. Ibid.

12. Cynthia L. Ogden, et al., "Prevalence and Trends in Overweight Among US Children and Adolescents, 1999–2000," *JAMA*, 288, no. 14 (October 9, 2002): 1728–32. "Overweight" among children was defined as "at or above the 95th percentile of body mass index (BMI: calculated as weight in kilograms divided by the square of height in meters) for age. At risk for overweight is defined as at or above the 85th percentile of BMI for age."

13. Salynn Boyles, "Supersized Kids, Diminishing Health," WebMD Feature, December 11, 2001, http://aolsvc.health.webmd.aol.com/content/Article/13/3606_1052.htm?printing=true.

14. Jeanie Lerche Davis, "Childhood Obesity Seen Even in Preschool," *Web MD Medical News*, May 5, 2003, http://my.webmd.com/content/Article/64/72383.htm?printing=true.

15. Sarah Yang, "San Diego Conference Tackles Child Obesity Epidemic," press release from UC Berkeley, January 2, 2003, http://www.berkeley.edu/news/media/releases/2003/01/02_obesity.html.

16. "Parents Unaware of Danger of Fat Children," Reuters Health, June 5, 2004.

17. Amy Norton, "Teen Obesity Tied to Adult Death Risk," Sandia National Laboratories, January 20, 2004, http://www.sandia.gov/health/update/20040120elin002.html.

18. Kevin R. Fontaine, et. al., "Years of Life Lost Due to Obesity," *JAMA* 289, no. 2 (January 8, 2003): 187–93.

19. Jeffrey B. Schwimmer, Tasha M. Burwinkle, and James W. Varni, "Health-Related Quality of Life of Severely Obese Children and Adolescents," *JAMA* 289, no. 14 (April 9, 2003): 1813.

20. J. J. Reilly, et al., "Health Consequences of Obesity," www.archdischild.com.

21. Ibid.

22. Ralph Winter, "Reconsecration to a Wartime, not a Peacetime, Lifestyle," in *Perspectives on the World Christian Movement,* ed. Ralph Winter and Steven Hawthorne (Pasadena, CA.: William Carey Library, 1981), 814.

23. Ibid.

24. "Heavy Kids More Likely to Bully, Be Bullied," Reuters Health, May 3, 2004.

25. Ibid.

26. *New England Journal of Medicine* 350 (2004): 2362–74.

27. "Arteries Already Stiff in Obese 7-Year-Old Children," Reuters Health, September 27, 2004.

28. "Obesity Can Cause Heart Attacks in Kids," Reuters Health, June 30, 2004.

29. *Pediatrics,* 2001:107.

30. "Childhood Obesity a Serious Problem," May 1, 2002, CBSNews.com.

31. *Archives of Disease in Childhood,* December 2002.

32. M. Fusco, "Bariatric Surgery: Do the Benefits Outweigh the Risks?" *Healthcare Risk Manager* 10, no. 22 (2004): 1–3, http://www.magmutual .com/mmic/articles/2004_Q1.pdf.

33. *International Journal of Cancer,* November 1, 2004, reported by Reuters Health, October 18, 2004.

34. *New England Journal of Medicine* 346, no. 16 (April 18, 2002).

35. Boyles, "Supersized Kids."

36. Ibid.

37. "'Shocking' Diabetes Prediction," June 14, 2003, CBSNews.com.

38. Arlene Dohm, "Gauging the Labor Force Effects of Retiring Baby-Boomers," *Monthly Labor Review,* July 2000, 17.

39. Ibid., 25.

40. Ibid.

41. Robert Brokamp, "Six Social Security Myths," Motley Fool, http://fool .com/news/commentary/2004/commentary040308RB.htm?source= mppromo.

42. David R. Francis, "A Brighter Outlook for Social Security," *Christian Science Monitor,* March 8, 2004, http://www.csmonitor.com/2004/0308/ p17s01-coop.html.

43. Tim Penny, "Social Security Needs Long-Term Overhaul, Not Campaign Slogans," *Christian Science Monitor,* March 15, 2004, http://www .csmonitor.com/2004/0315/p09s02-coop.html.

44. M. L. Davidlus, et al., "Relation of Body Mass Index in Young Adulthood and Middle Age to Medicare Expenditures in Older Age," *JAMA* 292, no. 22 (December 8, 2004): 2743–49.

Chapter 3

1. "Fat Americans Overwhelm Diagnostic Machines," Reuters News, December 1, 2004, www.reuters.com/newsArticle.jhtml?type=health News&storyID=6968823&section=news.

2. *JAMA,* 289 (2003): 450–53.

3. "Why Are We So Fat?" *National Geographic,* August 2004, 59.

4. *Pediatrics,* January 2004.

5. "Fast Food May Be Addictive, Say Scientists," www.abc.net.av/science/ news/health/HealthRepublish_773973.htm.

6. "You Won't Believe What Makes You Fat," June 1, 2004, www.member .compuserve.com/new/html/live/scoop/cs.13.html.

7. "Preventing Childhood Obesity: Health in the Balance; A Report of the Institute of Medicine" (National Academy Press, 2004), http://www.iom .edu/report.asp?id=22596.

8. "All It Takes Is Eight Minutes," Hispanic Magazine.com, June 2003.
9. http://www.kpvi.com/index.cfm?page=nbcstories.cfm&ID=2025.

Chapter 5

1. Steve Farkas, Jean Johnson, and Ann Duffett, "A Lot Easier Said Than Done: Parents Talk About Raising Children in Today's America; A Report from Public Agenda (New York, 2002), 20.
2. For more information on raising a child to be healthy physically, emotionally, relationally, and spiritually, see W. L. Larimore, A. Sorenson, and S. Sorenson, *The Highly Healthy Child* (Grand Rapids, MI: Zondervan Publishers, 2004), or W. L. Larimore, A. Sorenson, and S. Sorenson, *God's Design for the Highly Healthy Child* (Grand Rapids, MI: Zondervan Publishers, 2004), www.highlyhealthy.net.
3. K. K. Davison and L. L. Birch, "Childhood Overweight: A Contextual Model and Recommendations for Future Research," *Obesity Reviews* 2, no. 3 (August 2001): 159–71.
4. Ibid.
5. Steve Jordahl, "Obese Kids Lose Weight When Parents Help," *Family News in Focus*, August 15, 2003.
6. Jeanie Lerche Davis, "Childhood Obesity Seen Even in Preschool," May 5, 2003, http://www.webmd.com/content/Article/64/72383.htm.
7. Moria Golan and Abraham Weizman, "Familial Approach to the Treatment of Childhood Obesity: Conceptual Model," *Journal of Nutritional Education* 33, no. 2: 103.
8. Ibid.
9. Davison and Birch, "Childhood Overweight," *Obesity Reviews* 2, no. 3 (August 2001): 163.
10. Texas Children's Hospital, "Tips for Parents," www2.texaschildrens hospital.org/internetarticles/uploadedfiles/321.pdf.
11. Mozhdeh B. Bruss, Joseph Morris, and Linda Dannison, "Prevention of Childhood Obesity: Sociocultural and Familial Factors," *Journal of the American Dietetic Association* 103, no. 8 (August 2003): 1042.
12. Golan and Weizman, "Familial Approach," 105.
13. Richard J. Deckelbaum and Christine L. Williams, "Childhood Obesity: The Health Issue," *Obesity Research* 9, suppl. no. 4 (November 2001): 239S–42S.
14. Committee on Nutrition, "Prevention of Pediatric Overweight and Obesity," *Pediatrics* 112, no. 2 (August 2003): 425.
15. Bruss, Morris, and Dannison, "Prevention of Childhood Obesity," 1043.
16. Ibid.

17. Andrew M. Tershakovec and Kerri Kuppler, "Ethnicity, Insurance Type, and Follow-up in a Pediatric Weight Management Program," *Obesity Research* 11, no. 1 (January 2003): 19.

18. Valerie A. Long, "Families That Eat Together Are Healthier," University of New Hampshire Cooperative Extension, from an article posted on http://www.ceinfo.unh.edu/common/documents/gsc6101.htm.

19. Committee on Nutrition, "Prevention of Pediatric Overweight," 426.

20. "Want to Be a Good Parent? Do This!" August 18, 2002, http://member.compuserve.com/new/html/fte/2k/10.html.

21. Mimi Knight, "The Family That Eats Together . . . ," *Christian Parenting Today,* January/February 2002, http://www.christianitytoday.com/cpt/2002/001/3.30.html.

22. Committee on Nutrition, "Prevention of Pediatric Overweight," 425–26.

23. *International Journal of Obesity* 28, no. 7 (July 2004): 858–69.

24. Jennifer O. Fisher and Leann L. Birch, "Eating in the Absence of Hunger and Overweight in Girls from 5 to 7 Years of Age," *American Journal of Clinical Nutrition* 71 (2000): 1054–61.

25. Golan and Weizman, "Familial Approach," 102.

26. Shannon Brownlee, "Too Heavy, Too Young," *Time,* January 21, 2002, http://www.Time.com/time/covers/110102012/obesity.html.

27. "Helping Your Overweight Child," NIH Publication No. 03-4096, April 2003, http://www.niddk.nih.gov/health/nutrit/pubs/helpchld.htm.

28. Ibid.

29. H. G. Koenig, M. E. McCullough, and D. B. Larson, *Handbook of Religion and Health* (Oxford University Press, 2001).

30. Kenneth Ferraro, a professor of sociology and psychological sciences at Purdue University in West Lafayette, Indiana, has published a study that showed that religious participation is associated with higher body weight. His study of 3,600 people found that Southern Baptists are heaviest, with Jews, Muslims, and Buddhists less likely to be overweight (http://news.uns.purdue.edu/html4ever/9803.Ferraro.fat.html).

Ferraro says, ". . . overeating may be one sin that pastors and priests regularly overlook. And as such, many firm believers may have not-so-firm bodies." Ferraro says religion may curtail some of the unhealthful effects of being overweight. "What appears to be happening is a counterbalancing effect," he says. "Religious adults report higher levels of well-being. In general, obese persons are more likely to be depressed and dissatisfied with their health, but among religious persons, weight had no effect on well-being (http://news.uns.purdue.edu/html4ever/9803.Ferraro.fat. html).

Nevertheless, there is evidence of the harm of obesity among faith communities. In one example, the Annuity Board of the Southern Baptist

Convention in Dallas reported that the top two medical claims paid by the denomination's health insurance program in 2002 were for obesity-related ailments: back problems and high blood pressure (http://www .religionwriters.com/public/tips/061404/061404c.shtml).

31. I. Springer, "And Now . . . The Jewish Diet," Jewz.com, February 17, 2005, http://www.jewz.com/Artandent/aande.php?text=now_jewish_ diet.txt. "Weight Management During the Jewish Holidays," MedicineNet.com, October 23, 2002, http://www.medicinenet.com/script/main/art.asp? articlekey=21254. K. Burns, "Muslims and Weight Loss," Islam Online, October 5, 2000, http://www.islamonline.net/iol-english/dowalia/techng-2000-oct-07/techng4.asp.

32. "Beware! The No. 1 Diet Saboteur," December 16, 2003, http://member .compuserve.com/homerealestate/package.jsp?name=f . . .

33. Bruss, Morris, and Dannison, "Prevention of Childhood Obesity," 1042–45.

34. Ellen Hale, "Junk Food Super-Sizing Europeans," *USA Today,* November 18, 2003, 14A.

Chapter 6

1. "Gaining Weight? Blame Your Bedtime," Netscape News, July 31, 2003, www.defeatdiabetes.org/Articles'weight030731.htm.

2. M. Sekine, et al., "A Dose-Response Relationship Between Short Sleeping Hours and Childhood Obesity: Results of the Toyama Birth Cohort Study," *Child Care Health Development* 28, no. 2 (March 2002): 163–70, www.ncbi.nlm.nih.gov/entrez/query.fcgi?cmd=Retrieve&db=PubMed &dopt=Citation.

3. R. von Kreis, et al., "Reduced Risk for Overweight and Obesity in 5- and 6-Year-Old Children by Duration of Sleep: A Cross-Sectional Study," *International Journal of Obesity* 26 (2002): 710–16.

4. "Most U.S. Families Have This Big Problem," March 30, 2004, http://member.compuserve.com/new/html/live/scoop/cs/2.html.

5. *NSF Alert,* January 8, 2003, www.sleepfoundation.org/Alert/alert010803 .cfm.

6. "Guess What 17% of Teens Do at 2 a.m.?" June 14, 2004, http://member .compuserve.com/new/html/live/scoop/cs/17.html.

7. "Can You Sleep Off Fat?" November 18, 2004, www.cbsnews.com/ stories/2004/11/16/health/printable656062.shtml.

8. "What Happens If You Don't Sleep Enough?" March 30, 2004, http:// member.compuserve.com/news/package.jsp?name=news/sleep.

9. "Best Reason Yet to Sleep in Late," November 22, 2003, http://member .compuserve.com/new/html/live/scoop/cs/4.html.

10. "Study Links Sleep Loss to Teens' Suicide Behaviors," Reuters News, October 22, 2004. Story based on X. Liu, "Sleep and Adolescent Suicide Behavior," *Sleep* 27, no. 7 (November 2004): 1351–58.
11. Steve Farkas, Jean Johnson, and Ann Duffett, "A Lot Easier Said Than Done: Parents Talk About Raising Children in Today's America; A Report from Public Agenda" (New York, 2002), 13.
12. Federal Trade Commission, "Children as Consumers of Entertainment Media: Media Usage, Marketing Behavior and Influences, and Ratings Effects," September 1, 2000.

Chapter 7

1. *Resource Guide for Nutrition and Physical Activity Interventions to Prevent Obesity and Other Chronic Diseases,* Department of Health and Human Services, Centers for Disease Control and Prevention, Nutrition, Physical Activity, and Obesity Prevention Program, Attachment 7, "Reduce Television Time in Children," 37.
2. "For Every Two Hours of TV You Watch . . . ," *CompuServe News,* July 1, 2004, http://member.compuserve.com/news/package.jsp?name=news/watch, reporting on a study published in the *Journal of the American Medical Association.*
3. *International Journal of Obesity* 27 (2003): 827–33.
4. "Bizarre Physical Effect of Watching TV," July 1, 2004, http://member.compuserve.com/new/html/live/scoop/cs/19html, based on a report from BBC News Online.
5. "Too Much TV in Childhood Tied to Poor Health Later," Reuters Health, July 16, 2004, reporting on a study published in *Lancet.*
6. "Too Much TV Linked to High Cholesterol in Kids," Associated Press, November 13, 1990.
7. *Seven Shocking Reasons to Watch What Kids Watch: How TV Affects Children* (Broadman and Holman Publishers, 1996), www.christiananswers.net/tv1/tvb-ch5.html.
8. "Kids Who Watch More TV Eat Fewer Vegetables—Study," Reuters, December 8, 2003, reporting on a study published in *Pediatrics.*
9. "Kids Do Much of Their Munching in Front of TV," Reuters Health, July 2, 2004, based on an article in the *American Journal of Clinical Nutrition,* June 2004.
10. "U.S. Panel: Childhood Obesity a National Crisis," Reuters Health, September 30, 2004.
11. "Television Ads Promoting Unhealthy Food for Children," AAP Newsfeed, August 2, 2001.

12. "TV, Eating Out Makes Kids Fat, Studies Agree," Reuters, February 24, 2004.

13. Joan Ryan, "Planet Twinkie and the Junk-Food Assault on Our Kids," *Bergen County Record,* May 30, 2002, www.commercialalert.org/planettwinkie.htm.

14. Jennifer Warner, "Video Games, TV Double Childhood Obesity Risk," *WebMD Weight Loss Clinic Medical News,* July 2, 2004, reporting on an article in *Obesity Research,* June 2004.

15. Chelsea Stark, "UT Study Links Games, Obesity," March 26, 2004, www.dailytexanonline.com/news/2004/03/26/University/Ut.Study.Links .Games.Obesity-642619.shtml.

16. "Television Viewing and Television in Bedroom Associated with Over-weight Risk Among Low-Income Preschool Children," *Pediatrics* 109 (2002): 1028–35.

17. Barbara J. Brock, "TV Free Families: Are They Lola Granolas, Normal Joes or High and Holy Snots?" http://www.tvturnoff.org/brock1.htm.

18. Ibid., "Question 2: What Do They Do with All That Free Time?" http://www.tvturnoff.org/brock2.htm.

19. Ibid.

20. Barbara J. Brock, "TV Free Families: Are They Lola Granolas, Normal Joes or High and Holy Snots? Question 4: Do They Substitute Com-puter and Internet Use for TV?" http://www.tvturnoff.org/brock4.htm.

21. "TV, Eating Out Makes Kids Fat," Reuters, February 24, 2004.

Chapter 8

1. See www.medbroadcast.com.

2. Kathleen Doheny, "It's Never Too Early to Teach Kids the Activity Habit," *USA Today,* November 5, 2004.

3. Ibid.

4. "The No. 1 Excuse for Not Exercising," June 2, 2004, http://member .compuserve.com/new/html/live/scoop/cs/18.html.

5. "Music = Exercise = an Odd Side Effect," March 3, 2004, http://member/ compuserve.com, from a study published in *Heart & Lung.*

6. "The Best Exercise for Weight Loss," June 1, 2004, http://member. compuserve.com/new/html/live/scoop/cs/11.html, reporting a study that appeared in *Medicine & Science in Sports & Exercise.*

7. "Do This: Never Gain Another Pound," March 5, 2004, http://member .compuserve.com/new/html/live/scoop/cs/17.html, reporting on a story in *USA Today.*

8. Originally published in the *Archives of Internal Medicine.*

9. Ganley T. Sherman C: "Exercise and Children's Health: A Little Counseling Can Pay Lasting Dividends." *The Physician and Sports Medicine* 2000; 28(2): 85–92.

Chapter 9

1. Betsy McCormack, *Fit Over 40 for Dummies* (Foster City, CA.: IDG Books Worldwide, 2001), 59.
2. Sally Squires, "Overfed, Undernourished," *Washington Post,* September 21, 2004, HE01, http://www.washingtonpost.com/wp-dyn/articles/A36955-2004Sep20.html. Based upon the report of the Dietary Guidelines Scientific Advisory Committee, which can be found at http://www.health.gov/dietaryguidelines.
3. P. A. Quatromoni, D. L. Copenhafer, R. B. D'Agostino, and B. E. Millen, "Dietary Patterns Predict the Development of Overweight in Women: The Framingham Nutrition Studies," *Journal of the American Dietetic Association* 102, no. 9 (2002): 1239–46.
4. *American Journal of Preventive Health,* October 16, 2004.
5. "1% or Less Campaigns," Center for Science in the Public Interest, http://cspinet.org/nutrition/1less.htm.
6. "School Milk Makes the Grade: Student Nutritional Status Improves with Enhanced Milk Product," National Dairy Council, 2002.
7. *Obesity Research,* April 2004.
8. B. A. Dennison, H. L. Rockwell, and S. L. Baker, "Excess Fruit Juice Consumption by Preschool-Aged Children Is Associated with Short Stature and Obesity," *Pediatrics* 99 (1997): 15–22.
9. *Journal of the American Dietetic Association* 104, no. 4 (April 2004): 664.
10. Walter C. Willett and P. J. Skerrett, *Eat, Drink, and Be Healthy: The Harvard Medical School Guide to Healthy Eating* (Fireside, 2002).

Chapter 10

1. *Journal of the American Dietetic Association* 103, no. 11 (November 2003): 1541–56.
2. Steve Jordahl, "Obese Kids Lose Weight When Parents Help," *Family News in Focus,* August 15, 2003.
3. *Journal of the American Dietetic Association* 104, no. 7 (July 2004): 1076–79.
4. Steve Farkas, Jean Johnson, and Ann Duffett, "A Lot Easier Said Than Done: Parents Talk About Raising Children in Today's America; A Report from Public Agenda" (New York, 2002), 20.

5. Ibid., 17.
6. *American Journal of Epidemiology,* July 2003.
7. *Journal of the American Dietetic Association* 103, no. 12 (December 2003).
8. *American Journal of Clinical Nutrition* 50 (1989): 1303–7. *FASEB Journal* 13 (1999): A871.
9. P. Zollo, *Wise Up to Teens: Insights into Marketing and Advertising to Teenagers,* 2nd ed. (Ithaca, NY: New Strategist Publications, 1999).
10. D. Neumark-Sztainer, M. Story, D. Ackard, et al., "The 'Family Meal': Views of Adolescents," *Journal of Nutritional Education* 32 (2000): 329–34; Matthew W. Gillman, Sheryl L. Rifas-Shiman, A. Lindsay Frazier, et al., "Family Dinner and Diet Quality Among Older Children and Adolescents," *Archives of Family Medicine* 9 (2000): 235–40.
11. Ibid.
12. Neumark-Sztainer, "Family Meal."
13. Gillman, "Family Dinner"; D. Neumark-Sztainer, P. J. Hannan, M. Story, et al., "Family Meal Patterns: Associations with Sociodemographic Characteristics and Improved Dietary Intake Among Adolescents," *Journal of the American Dietetic Association* 103 (2003): 317–22.
14. Marla E. Eisenberg, Rachel E. Olson, Dianne Neumark-Sztainer, et al., "Correlations Between Family Meals and Psychosocial Well-Being Among Adolescents," *Archives of Pediatric and Adolescent Medicine* 158 (2004): 792–96.
15. "Dietary Guidance for Healthy Children Aged 2 to 11 Years," *Journal of the American Dietetic Association* 104 (2004): 660–77; L. Jahns, A. M. Siega-Riz, B. M. Popkin, "The Increasing Prevalence of Snacking Among U.S. Children from 1977 to 1996," *Journal of Pediatrics* 138 (2001): 493–98.

Chapter 11

1. J. F. Bogden, *Fit, Healthy, and Ready to Learn: A School Health Policy Guide* (Alexandria, VA: National Association of State Boards of Education [NASBE], 2000). Action for Healthy Kids, "The Role of Sound Nutrition and Physical Activity in Academic Achievement," 2004, http://www.actionforhealthykids.org/docs/fs_npaa.pdf.
2. "Preventing Childhood Obesity: Health in the Balance; A Report of the Institute of Medicine" (National Academy Press, 2004), http://www.iom.edu/report.asp?id=22596.
3. S. Schoenthaler, "Abstracts of Early Papers on the Effects of Vitamin-Mineral Supplementation on IQ and Behavior," *Personality and Individ-*

ual Differences 12, no. 4 (1991): 343. S. Schoenthaler, et al., "Controlled Trial of Vitamin-Mineral Supplementation: Effects on Intelligence and Performance," *Personality and Individual Differences* 12, no. 4 (1991): 361.

4. American School Food Service Association (ASFSA), "Impact of Hunger and Malnutrition on Student Achievement," *School Board Food Service Research Review,* Spring 1989, 17–21.

5. Center on Hunger, Poverty, and Nutrition Policy, *Statement on the Link Between Nutrition and Cognitive Development in Children* (Medford, MA: Tufts University School of Nutrition, 1995).

6. T. Harper, "The New PE," *Sky Magazine,* September 2004, 88–90.

7. National Association for Sport and Physical Education (NASPE), Executive Summary, *Shape of the Nation,* 2001. R. J. Shephard, et al., "Required Physical Activity and Academic Grades: A Controlled Longitudinal Study," in *Children and Sport,*" ed. Limarinen and Valimaki (Berlin: Springer-Verlag, 1984), 58–63; NASPE, "New Study Supports Physically Fit Kids Perform Better Academically," 2002.

8. R. J. Shephard, "Curricular Physical Activity and Academic Performance," *Pediatric Exercise Science* 9 (1997): 113–26.

9. C. W. Symons, et al., "Bridging Student Health Risks and Academic Achievement Through Comprehensive School Health Programs," *Journal of School Health* 67, no. 6 (1997): 220–27.

10. Centers for Disease Control and Prevention, Youth Risk Behavior Survey, 1995.

11. International Life Sciences Institute, "Improving Children's Health Through Physical Activity: A New Opportunity; A Survey of Parents and Children About Physical Activity Patterns," July 1997.

12. "Public Attitudes Toward Physical Education: Are Schools Providing What the Public Wants? A Survey Conducted by Opinion Research Corporation International of Princeton, NJ, for the National Association for Sport and Physical Education," http://www.aahperd.org/naspe/pdf_files/survey_public.pdf.

13. Harper, "The New PE."

14. Our list is adapted from "Ten Steps to Bringing Healthier Foods into Schools," Stonyfield Farm, http://stonyfield.com/MenuForChange/ParentActionKit/BringingHealthierFoodsIntoSchools.cfm.

15. Assessing both the nutritional and the physical activity environments at your child's school:

   ■ *Assessing Your Child's School,* http://208.142.197.5/hkn/word_docs/assessing_your_school.doc. This tool, developed by the American Cancer Society and Healthy Schools–Healthy Kids Initiative, is a

fifteen-question survey to assess the health education and environment in your school (including nutrition and physical activity).

- *School Health Index,* http://apps.nccd.cdc.gov/shi/. The CDC designed
  this tool to allow parents, teachers, and school officials to assess the
  strengths and weaknesses of health promotion policies and programs
  as they relate to nutrition, physical activity, and tobacco use. The tool
  has scorecards you can use for elementary schools or middle/high
  schools. After completing the assessment of your child's school, you
  can use this tool to develop an action plan for improving school
  health. There are also hyperlinks to many useful resources for school
  health and safety.

Assessing the nutritional environment at your child's school:

- *Changing the Scene: Improving the School Nutrition Environment,*
  http://www.fns.usda.gov/tn/Resources/changing.html. This tool, developed by the USDA, allows parents, teachers, administrators, and others
  to identify areas needing improvement in their school nutrition and
  food service.
- *Menu for Change—assessment questions,* http://stonyfield.com/
  MenuForChange/StepsForPilotProgram.cfm. This twelve-question
  assessment form from Stonyfield Farm will help you evaluate the
  food-service and nutrition policies in your child's school.

Assessing the physical activity environment at your child's school:

- *Is Your Child's Physical Education Program Ready to Prevent Obesity?*
  http://www.aahperd.org/naspe/template.cfm?template=prevent.html.
  This assessment tool, with ten questions to evaluate strengths and
  weaknesses of your school's PE program, was developed by the
  National Association for Sport and Physical Education.

16. A. Anderson, "Fitness Is Fun at Friendship Elementary," WNEG News,
    Channel 32, Toccoa, GA, February 16, 2005, http://www.wneg32.com/
    servlet/Satellite?pagename=WNEG/MGArticle/NEG_BasicArticle&c=
    MGArticle&cid=1031780860791&path=.
17. http://www.fns.usda.gov/tn/Resources/CalltoAction.pdf.
18. "Preventing Childhood Obesity: Health in the Balance; A Report of the
    Institute of Medicine," National Academy Press, 2004, http://www.iom.
    edu/report.asp?id=22596.
19. http://www.publichealthadvocacy.org/legislation/Healthy%20Bever-
    age%20Resolution.pdf.

20. Harper, "The New PE."
21. Ibid.
22. http://www.aahperd.org/naspe/template.cfm?template=prevent.html.

Chapter 12

1. www.cpgi.net/76tons. It's still in operation!
2. "Phat Times in Philly: City Moves to Lose Weight," CNN.com, July 3, 2001, http://archives.cnn.com/2001;HEALTH/diet.fitness/07/03/philly .weight.
3. "Philadelphia Looks to Shed Pounds, Reputation," Associated Press, July 2, 2001, www.usatoday.com/news/health/2001-07-02-philly.htm.
4. http://healthhighlights.ihc.com/article.asp?page=50.
5. R. Giordano, "The Target Age: Preteens to Middle Schoolers; Health Clubs Moving Fast to Help 'Tweens' Shape Up," *Philadelphia Inquirer,* February 2, 2004, http://www.philly.com/mld/inquirer/7852387.htm.
6. You can get more information about the American Cancer Society's Generation Fit Action Packet at our Web site (www.SuperSizedKids. com), or you can contact your local American Cancer Society or call 1-800-ACS-2345.
7. American Cancer Society Recommendation for Community Action, http://www.cancer.org/docroot/PED/content/PED_3_2X_Community_ Action_Needed_for_Healthful_Lifestyles.asp.
8. "Preventing Childhood Obesity: Health in the Balance; A Report of the Institute of Medicine" (National Academy Press, 2004), http://www.iom .edu/report.asp?id=22596.
9. Kidwalk-to-School, Department of Health Services, Centers for Disease Control and Prevention, 2000.
10. http://www.nhtsa.dot.gov/people/injury/pedbimot/bike/saferouteshtml /overview.html#1.
11. "Matthew Brown Act Becomes Law," http://www.runningnetworkarchives. com/runnertriathletenews/news/mba_law2001.html.
12. "T.A. Bronx Program Shows Way," *T.A. Magazine,* Spring 2004, 11, http://www.saferoutestoschool.org/.
13. "Philadelphia Looks to Shed Pounds, Reputation."

Chapter 13

1. "The Three States with the Fattest People," October 29, 2003, http:// member.compuserve.com/new/html/live/scoop/cs/12.html.

2. Robert Tanner, "States Look to Combat Obesity with Laws," Associated Press, December 22, 2003, http://member.compuserve.com/news/story. jsp?oldflok=FF-APO-1 . . .

3. K. Edwards, "Ad-dicted Kids," *Kennebec (Augusta, ME) Journal*, December 2, 2004, http://kennebecjournal.mainetoday.com/news/local/1187551. shtml.

4. "Diet, Nutrition and the Prevention of Chronic Diseases: Report of a Joint WHO/FAO Expert Consultation," WHO Technical Report Series, no. 916 (Geneva: World Health Organization, 2003).

5. G. Hastings, et al., *Review of Research on the Effects of Food Promotion to Children* (Glasgow: University of Strathclyde, Centre for Social Marketing, 2003), http://www.foodstandards.gov.uk/news/pressreleases/ foodtochildren.

6. "Pestering Parents Report: How Food Companies Market Obesity to Children," Center for Science in the Public Interest, November 10, 2003, http://cspinet.org/new/pdf/pesteringparentsnopictures.pdf.

7. "CSPI Hits Marketing Junk Food to Kids," http://cspinet.org/new/ 200311101.html.

8. "Pestering Parents Report."

9. U.S. Department of Health and Human Services, Centers for Disease Control and Prevention, National Center for Health Statistics, *Healthy People 2000 Final Review*, DHHS Publication no. 01-0256 (Hyattsville, MD, 2001).

10. S. Y. Kim, R. M. Nayga, and O. Capps, "The Effect of Food Label Use on Nutrient Intakes: An Endogenous Switching Regression Analysis," *Journal of Agricultural and Resource Economics* 25 (2000): 215–31.

11. A. S. Levy and B. M. Derby, *The Impact of the NLEA on Consumers: Recent Findings from FDA's Food Label and Nutrition Tracking System* (Washington, DC: Center for Food Safety and Applied Nutrition, U.S. Food and Drug Administration, 1996).

12. U.S. Department of Health and Human Services, Food and Drug Administration, *Federal Register* 64 (1999): 62772–74.

13. S. Crutchfield, F. Kuchler, and J. N. Variyam, "The Economic Benefits of Nutrition Labeling: A Case Study for Fresh Meat and Poultry Products," *Journal of Consumer Policy* 24 (2001): 185–207.

14. "Preventing Childhood Obesity: Health in the Balance; A Report of the Institute of Medicine" (National Academy Press, 2004), http://www.iom .edu/report.asp?id=22596.

15. J. Meikle, S. Boseley, and F. Lawrence, "Agenda for a Healthy Nation, but Will It Work?" *Guardian* (London), November 17, 2004, http://www .guardian.co.uk/smoking/Story/0,2763,1352969,00.html.

16. Ibid.

17. B. Gardiner, "Panel Recommends Changes to Fight Obesity," Associated Press (London), May 29, 2004, http://www.defeatdiabetes.org/Articles/obesity2040529.htm.

18. Ibid.

19. B. A. Almanza, D. Nelson, and S. Chai, "Obstacles to Nutrition Labeling in Restaurants," *Journal of the American Dietetic Association* 97 (1997): 157–61.

20. Ibid.

21. R. Milich, J. Anderson, and M. Mills, "Effects of Visual Presentation of Caloric Values on Food Buying by Normal and Obese Persons," *Perceptual and Motor Skills* 42 (1976): 155–62.

22. Heart Institute of Spokane, Menu2 Pilot Results, http://www.this.org./comm_edu/mn2rest.html.

23. "Preventing Childhood Obesity."

24. CDE and Child Nutrition Section, "Better Breakfast, Better Learning," Washington State Office of Superintendent of Public Instruction, 1994.

25. See our list on our Web site at www.SuperSizedKids.com, http://cspinet.org/nutritionpolicy/gastaxrestrictions.pdf.

26. "CSPI Hits Marketing Junk Food to Kids," http://cspinet.org/new/200311101.html.

27. M. Nestle and M. F. Jacobson, "Halting the Obesity Epidemic: A Public Health Policy Approach," *Public Health Reports* 115 (January/February 2000): 12–24, http://www.cspinet.org/reports/obesity.pdf.

28. "CDC Urged to Rein in Obesity Now," Reuters News, October 20, 2004.

29. "Food Marketing and the Diets of Children and Youth," Institute of Medicine Food and Nutrition Board, October 14, 2004, http://www.iom.edu/project.asp?id=21939.

30. "Obesity-Drug Maker in Pact with Merck," Moneyline, *USA Today,* September 28, 2004, B1.

31. "Scientists Still Looking for Fat-Fighting Pill," Reuters, June 4, 2004, www.msnbc.msn.com/id/5138454/.

32. Daniel Q. Haney, "New Pill Helps with Smoking and Weight," Associated Press, March 10, 2004, www.uc.edu/news/NR.asp?id=1417.

33. Ibid.

34. Steve Connor and Jeremy Laurance, "Fat Chance: How the Wonder Drug to Curb Obesity Turned Out to Be an Apparition," July 19, 2004, http://news.independent.co.uk/uk/health_medical/story.jsp?story=542410.

35. "CDC Urged to Rein in Obesity Now."

Appendix A

1. B. A. Dennison, H. L. Rockwell, and S. L. Baker, "Excess Fruit Juice Consumption by Preschool-Aged Children Is Associated with Short Stature and Obesity," *Pediatrics* 99 (1997): 15–22.
2. We do so because the 95th percentile (1) corresponds to a BMI of 30, which is the marker for obesity in adults (the 85th percentile corresponds to the overweight reference point for adults, which is a BMI of 25), (2) is recommended as a marker for children and adolescents to have an in-depth medical assessment, (3) identifies children that are very likely to have obesity persist into adulthood, (4) is associated with elevated blood pressure and lipids in older adolescents, and increases their risk of diseases, (5) is a criterion for more aggressive treatment, and (6) is a criterion in clinical research trials of childhood obesity treatments. http://www.obesity.org/subs/childhood/prevalence.shtml.

ABOUT THE AUTHORS

Walt Larimore, M.D., is one of America's best-known family physicians and is listed in the *Best Doctors in America, Who's Who in Medicine and Health-care,* and the *International Health Professionals of the Year*. His M.D. degree is from Louisiana State University and his Family Medicine residency was at Duke. He practiced four years in the Smoky Mountains before moving to Central Florida to practice for sixteen years. In 1996 he was named America's Outstanding Family Medicine Educator by the American Academy of Family Physicians. Dr. Larimore is now a full-time author and medical journalist. From 1996 to 2001, Dr. Larimore hosted over 850 daily episodes of the live *Ask the Family Doctor* show on Fox's *Health Network*—being awarded the prestigious Gracie Award by the American Women in Radio and Television. From 2002 to 2004, he hosted the *Focus on Your Family's Health* syndicated radio and TV features. He is a frequent guest on a wide variety of television and radio programs, including *The Today Show,* CBS's *Morning Show,* several Fox News programs, and CNN. Dr. Larimore has published over 500 articles in dozens of medical and lay publications. He is also the author of more than a dozen books, including the bestsellers *Bryson City Tales: Stories of a Doctor's Practice in the Smoky Mountains* and *Alternative Medicine: The Christian Handbook*. His most recent books include *Why ADHD Doesn't Mean Disaster, God's Design for the Highly Healthy Child, God's Design for the Highly Healthy Teen,* and *God's Design for the Highly Healthy Person*. His Web site is www.DrWalt.com.

Sherri Flynt received her master's in public health from Loma Linda University. She is a registered and licensed dietitian and serves as head of the Center for Nutritional Excellence at Florida Hospital.

ABOUT FLORIDA HOSPITAL

For nearly one hundred years the mission of Florida Hospital has been to help our patients, guests, and friends achieve whole-person health and healing. With seven hospital campuses and fourteen walk-in medical centers, Florida Hospital cares for nearly one million patients every year.

Over a decade ago Florida Hospital began working with the Disney Corporation to create a groundbreaking facility that would showcase the model of healthcare for the twenty-first century and stay on the cutting edge of medical technology as it develops. Working with a team of medical experts, industry leaders, and health care futurists, we designed and built a whole-person health hospital named Celebration Health located in Disney's town of Celebration, Florida. Since opening its doors in 1997, Celebration Health has been awarded the Premier Patient Services Innovator Award as "The Model for Healthcare Delivery in the Twenty-first Century."

When Dr. Lydia Parmele, the first female physician in the state of Florida, and her medical team opened our first health care facility in 1908, their goal was to create a healing environment where they not only treated illness, but also provided the support and education necessary to help patients achieve whole-person health mentally, physically, spiritually, emotionally, and socially.

The lifestyle advocated by our founders remains central to all we do at Florida Hospital. We teach patients how to reduce the risk of disease through healthy lifestyle choices, encouraging the use of natural remedies such as fresh air, sunshine, water, rest, nutrition, exercise, outlook, faith, and interpersonal relationships.

Today, Florida Hospital:

- Ranks number one in the nation for inpatient admissions by the American Hospital Association
- Is the largest provider of Medicare services in the country
- Performs the most heart procedures each year, making it the No. 1 hospital fighting America's No. 1 killer—heart disease
- Operates many nationally recognized centers of excellence, including Cardiology, Cancer, Orthopedics, Neurology and Neurosurgery, Digestive Disorders and Minimally Invasive Surgery.
- Is one of the "Top 10 Best Places in the Country to Have a Baby," according to *Fit Pregnancy* magazine

For more information about Florida Hospital and our other whole-person health products, including books, music, videos, conferences, seminars, and other resources, please contact us at:

Florida Hospital Publishing
683 Winyah Drive, Orlando, FL 32803
Phone: 407-303-7711   ■   Fax: 407-303-1818
Email: healthproducts@flhosp.org
www.FloridaHospital.com   ■   www.CreationHealth.com